P9-AOT-427

Color Energy Therapy

A Newly Emerging, Ancient Healing Modality

This innovative book presents new information, not previously introduced to the masses on the use of color energy healing involving not merely physically applied color, but energetically produced color.

This book includes:

What color energy is * The twelve major chakras * The 13 Rays of Creation * Grounding, protection, clearing and balancing techniques * Chakra balancing * Aura scanning, reading and merging * The Energy Transferal technique * Working with crystals * Working with herbs * Opening your channels for healing * The crystallization process * Opening the heart chakra. * The role of ego in healing * Removing psychic hooks * Working with the different color rays * Ley line connecting * Solar plexus tying * Color, sound and movement---your personal blueprint * Causal plane clearing and creation * Responsibility as a healer * Bursting Through Blocks technique * The origin of Creation * Connecting to the Source * Alchemy and the holographic universe * The black ray defined * Multidimensional chakra balancing and linking * Multiple universes linking * The hyperspace experience * The shadow self * Camouflaging energy * The out-of-body experience * Psychic surgery * Advanced Psi Arts * The Emerald Star * and much more!

Healing with the Rainbow Rays

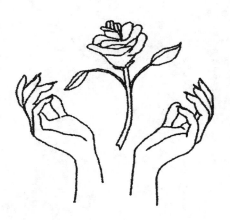

Healing with the Rainbow Rays

The Art of Color Energy Therapy

Alijandra

1995
Emerald Star Publishing
San Jose, California

Healing with the Rainbow Rays; The Art of Color Energy Therapy.
Copyright © 1995 by Alijandra.

Published by:
Emerald Star Publishing
P. O. Box 32818
San Jose, California 95152-2818

All rights reserved. No part of this book may be reproduced in any form without the expressed written consent of the publisher, except in the case of brief quotations embodied in critical articles and reviews.

The information presented in this book has been developed over many years of research, study and teaching by the author. However, this book is not intended to diagnose, prescribe or treat any physical or spiritual malady, nor is it intended in any way to be a replacement for medical or psychological consultation when needed. The author and publisher of this book do not guarantee the efficacy of any of the methods described. Only those who have successfully completed a "Rainbow Rays" certified instructor program are eligible to teach this material. Questions regarding permission to use this material for teaching purposes should be directed to the author in care of the publisher.

First Edition
First Printing, August 1995

Cover art: John Mason
Photography: Anthony Oliver
Illustrations: John Mason, James Marsh, and Sarah Steinbach
Book design and layout: Alijandra and Sarah Steinbach

Library of Congress Catalog Card Number: 95-90236

**Healing with the Rainbow Rays: The Art of Color Energy Therapy /
Alijandra**

ISBN 0-9645766-0-0
**1. Color Energy. 2. Self Help. 3. Metaphysical 4. Healing Arts
I. Alijandra II. Title**

Dedication

To my children, Tara and Kent,
for their support and patience.
To my love, Larry Smith,
for believing in me.
And always, Adassan.

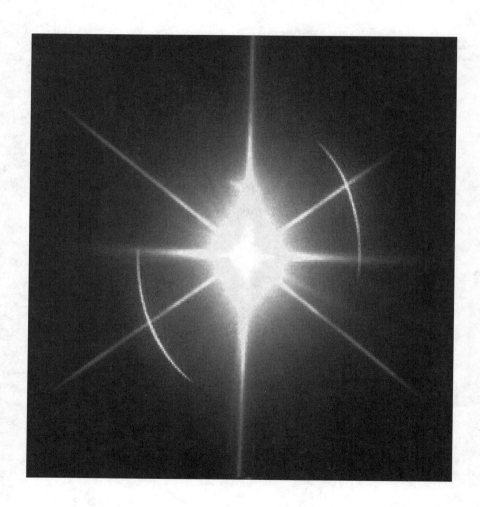

Acknowledgments

Healing With The Rainbow Rays is truly a group effort and there are many to thank:

First, I would like to acknowledge the wisdom and love of some of my multidimensional friends who work with me. Without them there would be no color healing data. They are LaLur, Adassan, Voltra, Hatonn, Korton, Mon-Ka, Althea, Saint Germain, Alana, Thor, Archangel Michael, Gaia, Elycia, Gossamer, Omega, and many more who have provided input to this work. I wish to thank the several people on this plane who, through the "channeling" process done in the consultation format, provided a vehicle for some of the data to come forth from the multidimensions.

My sincere appreciation goes to Dr. Frank Alper for the use of his material on opening and closing the aura, chakra balancing, and energy transferal. The information is contained within his book <u>Our Existence is Mind</u>.

Thank you, Ken Carey, for your permission to quote from your wonderful spiritual masterpiece (which I feel is destined to be a classic), <u>Starseed, The Third Millenium</u>.

I want to acknowledge visionary artist, John Mason, for knowing how to bring my vision into fruition.

My thanks to Bob Zelman, Ph.D., for the first go-around in the editing process. His editorial suggestions and personal spiritual evolution gave him a keen insight into how this book should be presented.

To my "soul-sister" Sandy Cline for her loving input, both editorial and supportive. She read every line of the work out loud(!), editing with razor-sharp clarity. She was my choice to provide the preface for this book, writing a beautiful, insightful piece.

Also, many thanks to Karen Lauer and Larry Smith for additional editing comments. They were much appreciated.

I owe a debt of gratitude to Sarah Steinbach for her tireless efforts doing book design and layout. I literally would have not been able to complete this work as easily, if at all, without her willingness to spend hours of extra time on it. As she so aptly put it, "It was like converting [my software] from horse and buggy to a diesel engine." There must have been times she just wished the manuscript would "drive" away!

There are several who assisted in a number of different areas: Jim Aldridge, Sandy Lewis, Jil Billingslea, Virginia Essene, Anthony Oliver, Christina (Chrissy) Feinstein, and DeeDee. You know how you helped. I love you all.

My love and appreciation to all of the class facilitators.

Table of Contents

Poems and Quotes

Foreword

For the one who is truly "open" there is nothing mysterious about the metaphysical nature inherent in ourselves and our everyday world. For the willing, intuition is the guide; straightforward as an arrow it leads each seeker past arcane and dated beliefs to the fantastic point where science and magic meet. *Healing with the Rainbow Rays* is a handbook for such a journey.

Alijandra reminds us that life's dark clouds are of our own making. Freedom from pain and suffering will not come from outside ourselves; it is up to us to slowly awaken to the damage we do, not only to each other, but to our beautiful Earth. It can be as simple as a spiteful thought, or as manifold as a murderous deed.

The techniques described in Alijandra's book offer a new way of "being," a fresh approach to healing the dull ache of humankind and the planet it exploits for its daily dose of pabulum.

Her unpretentious message focuses on remembering who we are and what we're to become. The subtext of her "lessons" supports the foundations of self-trust, the creative process, and the human need to explore beyond the five senses of one's world.

We must never forget that nature and poetry are one in the same; both are filled with structured meter, natural cadences, rhyme, and metaphor. Alijandra repeatedly alludes to the inseparability of man from the natural world we live in. As integral members of the cosmic order, we too become part of the universal song of the soul, made up of the radiant Rainbow Rays.

The last stanza of an ancient Inuit song goes:

> *And yet, there is only*
> *One Great Thing.*
> *The Only Thing.*
> *The Great Day that dawns,*
> *And the Light that fills the world.*

May the wondrous incandescence of the sacred rainbow rays shine upon you as you stand in a circled forest of blessings and reclaim your birthright ... a new Dawn has come.

Sandra Cline
Albuquerque, New Mexico
March, 1995

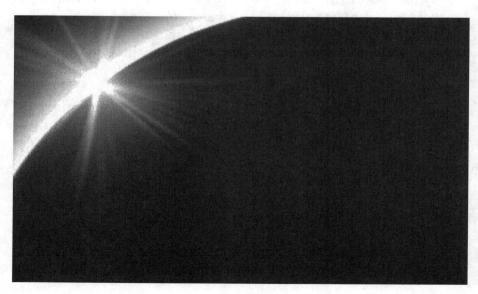

Introduction:

Starting the Adventure

Our purpose is to embody Spirit within our material bodies, to express universal Love and Light continuously, to create a blended, balanced, and unified mind-body connection, and to merge soul consciousness and physical consciousness into one new glorious being.

With the purchase of this book, you have entered a world of color! Open your heart and mind, put aside your preconceptions and illusions; be prepared to embark on a journey of discovery as you develop keen insight that can literally change your life for the better.

With your sixth senses of *perception* and *vision*, you will begin to notice how your home, this Earth, is composed of different frequencies of color. Some appear very solid, other aspects seem more ethereal, less substantive than your current level of perception. You will begin to find that these intensities of light are part of, yet distinguished from physical "reality", and that you can change this so-called reality through the use of color light energy.

Choosing this book wasn't a coincidence. Something led you to this subject. Perhaps, it was curiosity, a need to explore alternative healing modalities, or a desire to grow and empower yourself.

Whatever the reason, my sincere wish is that the following lessons provide a trigger to your growth process. The many color energy exercises can be used successfully for your own spiritual evolvement.

My goal is to facilitate others as they cope with the personal and universal planetary changes we are currently experiencing. Color healing work has come forth from the Source to help people clear and balance the physical, emotional, and mental parts of themselves, and align their spiritual selves with their other "bodies" or aspects. At a planetary level, color energy provides the opportunity for our planet to rebalance itself.

Many of the following chapters deal with controversial subjects including my personal experiences of inter-dimensional realities, alchemy, and the creation of the Cosmos. Please do not let the "stretched" boundaries of linear thinking discourage you. You may fear the expansive nature of color energy therapy; you may think of it as being, as we say, too "woo-woo".

If you are a more traditional-minded caregiver in the healing arts or sciences, please consider giving these techniques a try in your work with your patients or clients. Regardless of your personal beliefs or philosophies, I know that you will begin to see subtle, or even dramatic, results with color therapy. **Color energy healing knows no particular religion or belief system**. It is compatible with all, except for those religions or belief systems that are dogmatic or limited. Unless you can hold an open mind and an open heart, this is not the book for you.

Color healing is an energy modality unlike any other; it is the music of the spheres, a method to be honored. At the deepest level, color healing connects you to alternate dimensions of reality, to multiple planes of existence, and to the origin of Creation Itself. Its format appears simple yet it can be extremely intense. However, I've never known anyone incapable of channeling color energy. I've observed its effectiveness in numerous situations, even when all other healing methods have failed.

Healing With The Rainbow Rays is drawn from the material presented in my on-going color energy classes. It is meant to be a vehicle for spreading the color energy method of healing, but not a substitute for the experiential, instructor-guided training. The value of intensive, hands-on training with multiple healing partners, under the skilled direction of a color energy certified instructor, cannot be underestimated. The transfer of wisdom and knowledge from an intuitive teacher can totally change your life. If you can personally take the color energy classes, you should arrange to do so for your own transformation and growth; there is much power and uplifted vibration within the group framework. If you can't physically attend a color healing class, this book is the next best thing.

When you practice the techniques in this book that involve a healing partner or partners, be sure that they too are studying the book and have an equal skill level to your own.

This book should also be read and studied in a linear sequence, as each chapter takes you to a deeper level of understanding. But, it should be *understood* non-linearly, allowing its transformative nature to help shift you to a synergistic, interdimensional perspective.

This is universal information that is available to anyone who has the skills, desire, and willingness to tune in. However, grounding it into the Earth plane in an articulated, physical format is the task I accepted. This required discipline and constant, daily effort to align my will with Universal Will. This seven year *dharma* ("right action") was a spiritual journey of enfoldment for me. For the steady effort and constant action by my s/Self, I celebrate! This is the gift from the universe to me, and my gift to you on the physical Earth plane. I offer it to you with great Love.

May this work be of as much value to you in your life-walk as it has been in mine.

I wish you rainbows of color!

Alijandra
San Jose, CA
March 1995

Chapter 1

Color and Healing

"As I come forth I've given to you the Rays of the Rainbow. The Rainbow is a symbol that was given unto man long ago by Its Radiance and began a symbol of great promise. The promise is eternal peace, eternal love, and it should surely reign supremely upon Earth... Know now that all those who are ready are becoming the Rainbow."

---Archangel Michael

Are You a Healer?

Did you ever think that by residing on this planet Earth at this particular time, that you have taken on the responsibility to help to heal it in some way? We may actively attempt to heal ourselves; we may even facilitate the healing process in others. However, how many of us are aware that we may unconsciously be attempting to rebalance the imbalances of our earth? Perhaps, you have done this by working for peace or for the environment, or by saving our wildlife.

To help heal the earth, you need to begin to heal yourself. The misalignments of the human race have unbalanced the planet on which we live. I fully believe that our Earth reflects the energy of the beings that live upon it, that the imbalances of nature reflect what is going on within each of us.

> *Your mission at this time is to heal yourself*
> *and then help heal the planet in some way.*

Perhaps you find yourself actually attracted to the therapeutically oriented, direct healing methods such as nursing or massage therapy or color energy therapy.

How do you know if you have a particular talent for *hands-on* healing? Some telltale signs may help you to determine this. You may have experienced some-or all-of these signs:

1) People come to you for advice or comfort when they are down emotionally or mentally;
2) People ask you for advice or expect that you will help them when they are experiencing physical pain;

3) After you have been with someone in need, they feel better but you may feel worse;
4) You feel drained after being in crowds, or sometimes even with just a few people;
5) Your hands frequently feel hotter or have electrical sensations, particularly if you're helping someone;
6) You even may feel strange waves of "energy" travel through your being, from the top of your head and down your arms, especially when you are helping someone;
7) You often feel "spacey," or ungrounded;
8) You have a problem with gaining too much weight, and your metabolism rate has more to do with this than overeating;
9) *Green* or *rose* are the colors that look best on you;
10) You have a fascination with the body and how it works, and/or a real interest in the healing arts.

If you are able to answer "yes" to at least 3 of these examples, you are probably an unconscious healer. So, how do you change from being an unconscious healer to a conscious healer?

This book will provide the answers. You will discover useful exercises in self-development and techniques for learning to heal yourself and facilitate others' healing.

By healing yourself and healing Earth, you evolve as an essence. This evolution eventually leads to enlightenment and advanced levels of illumination. The later chapters of this book delve deeper into advanced techniques to facilitate your journey into universal consciousness.

Whether you ultimately choose the road of being a professional color therapist, or branch off into another specialty such as massage, crystals, or Reiki, by working with the material in this book you will at least have had good training in a re-emerging, very ancient style of healing. (The use of color as a source of healing goes back to the old "mystery schools" in which our predecessors practiced alchemy.)

What is Color Healing?

It is possible, as healers, to tap into interdimensional realms of consciousness. We call the source of this collective consciousness by many names: God, Allah, Jehovah, Great Spirit, or the Creator to name a few. As metaphysicians, or spiritually focused seekers, we see that the universe is not necessarily composed in a linear format, with everything in a neat little row of past, present, and future.

The color therapist sees the universe as a hologram; as a multi-faceted gem. The color energy healer views the person he/she is working with in a "wholistic", holographic way. *

The color therapist utilizing light energy, which emanates from this Source, is reflective of the full color spectrum. Color is *frequency of light*. Each color hue and shade vibrate on a specific frequency. Certain rays of color, or "laser light energy", can be used not only for enlightenment, attunement, and communication with intelligences beyond our five senses, but also for healing the body, mind, and the emotions. Color therapy can align the spiritual essence of a being. Its multi-level source of emanation makes it one of the most powerful methods of healing. It does not strictly rely on physical methods of therapy.

On Earth's physical plane, color is known for its healing (or lack of healing) propensities. Color in the environ-

---

* See Chapter 19 for an in-depth look at the holographic universe.

ment has a subtle but definite effect upon the well-being of a person. There have been studies using specific colors in hospitals. **Mint green** was shown to be effective in operating rooms, facilitating more rapid post-operative healing. **Light blue** in the conference rooms allowed for greater communication in meetings. **Rose pink** in the psychiatric areas calmed down hyper, irrational patients.

The color of clothes you wear can also affect how you feel in your day to day life. Color in this planet on which we live (commonly known as the "3rd dimension") is considered *pigmented* color, not *radiant* color. There is a difference.

Color on the inner planes, also known as "Rays of the Rainbow", or the rays that radiate from the "etheric Rainbow Temples", are not as we know it on this physical plane. The etheric rainbow temples are non-physical in origin, wherein the spiritual intent or idea of the Source is set in place. These temples, in turn, give the blueprint for physical creation to manifest. There are multiple magnitudes of color emanations that we are not even aware of on Earth. *

Our physical eyes cannot see this radiant color. However, our inner psychic sight is capable of perceiving this luminous brilliance. These etheric rays of light, properly channeled, provide an intense healing experience. The energies of a person are uplifted and harmonized, and clarity is restored.

Much of its benefit and the degree of healing attained depends, of course, on how receptive or open the person is to the light. However, the client need not be a believer in order to gain a healing. Another consideration is how much past negative karma † and thinking he/she is will-

---

*See Chapter 17 for a more in-depth explanation.

† The universal law of balance, or cause and effect. What one sows, one reaps.

ing to release. The primary healer is always the individual needing therapy but a healing channel can be a facilitator or "jump-starter" (a term I am fond of using) for the client's own healing energies to awaken.

One does not, however, have to be in a state of extreme imbalance to benefit from color healing. No application of light is ever wasted. The more one is infused with light, the closer one is to the realization that he/she and the cosmic Light are one and the same.

The color therapist brings forth color for the purpose of sending it out to those in need of it. It is felt throughout the body as a wave of energy - a sensation of heat (either electrical or magnetic) as it travels through and out the hands, and often through the heart and solar plexus centers. As this is happening, it can be seen intuitively, or sensed subtly.

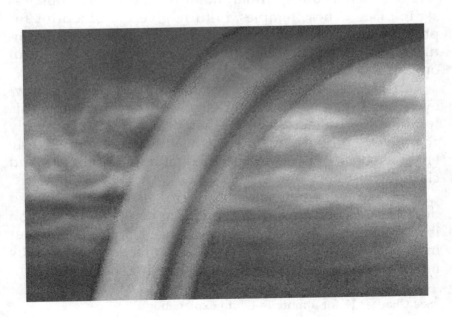

Chapter 2

Chakras and the Rays

Ten Thousand Lights

Ten thousand lights
running to and fro
Ten thousand lights
filled with worry and woe.

One small light
bringing joy and laughter,
One small light
all innocence and rapture.

One small light shining
with the heart of a child,
Transmutes 10,000 lights
filled with worry and guile.

---Korton
August 1991

The Twelve Major Chakras

Name	Color	Location	Organs/ Function
Physical Chakras			
First Chakra	Red	At base of spine	Bones, muscles, lower extremities
Second Chakra	Orange	Region of pelvic cavity. Between navel & base of spine	Reproductive organs, spleen balance
Third Chakra	Yellow	Abdominal region (navel)	Digestion, adrenal balance, ulcers
Emotional Chakras			
Fourth Chakra	Green/ Rose	Heart region	Heart and lungs, immune system, thymus balance
Fifth Chakra	Blue	Throat	Throat, upper bronchials, neurological thyroid balance
Mental/Spiritual Chakras			
Sixth Chakra	Indigo	Third eye, forehead	Pituitary gland, facial area (eyes, nose, ears)
Seventh Chakra	Purple	Crown of head	Brain area, pineal gland
Etheric Chakras			
Eighth Chakra	Silver	Below the feet approximately 6"	Feminine energy; grounds to earth
Ninth Chakra	Gold	Above the head approximately 6"	Masculine energy; connects to Source
Tenth Chakra	White	Palm chakra of dominant hand	Protection; contains all color
Eleventh Chakra	Clear	Palm chakra of non-dominant hand	Clarity and truth; contains all color
Twelfth Chakra	Black	Outside layer of auric field and approximately 12" below feet	Provides experiences for testing, energy movement, and grounding; contains all color

Chart 2-1

All living things have an electromagnetic field. What is it? It is the aura. The electric aspect of the aura is male or positive polarity. The magnetic aspect is female or negative polarity. The yin/yang symbol of the ancient Tao philosophy mirrors at a spiritual level what the male/ female electromagnetic energy reflects at a physical level-- "As above, so below."

When I refer to "negative" polarity for the female energy, I do not mean it in the bad or undesirable sense. The female yin energy is the receptive energy; the "cool" current in the Tao philosophy, which is enjoying a resurgence in popularity. The male energy is the yang, or positive polarity that transmits "warm" energy.

The aura reflects all aspects of the being. All emotions, thoughts, desires are reflected in the electromagnetic field. Shades and hues of color represent these emotions, thoughts, and desires. Darkened, dingy, or weak colors signify trouble areas wherever they are seen. People with visual intuitive abilities even can see symbols within this field. These symbols may be as common as the circle, star, and square, or as complicated as ancient script.

Our bodies contain a chakra system. A **chakra** is an energy center wherein a concentration of physical nerves congregate, overlaid by an energy "body" with subtler vibrations. The chakra is commonly referred to as a subtle wheel of energy. It is associated with a specific endocrine gland(s) or organ(s) in the physical body, and a consciousness in the emotional/mental bodies.

We have twelve[*] major chakras, seven within the body and five outside the body in the auric field. Most teachers of the chakra system teach that there are only seven or

---

[*] We technically have 13 chakras within our system if you count the two at the heart chakra. Since most people are used to referring to the throat chakra as the fifth, the 3rd eye as the sixth, and so forth, it seemed wisest to continue with that nomenclature.

nine centers of energy. I teach that there are twelve chakras with thirteen actual colors. The twelve major chakras form a rainbow. If you were to look only at the electromagnetic bodies of living beings, rather than their physical bodies, you would see a kaleidoscope of color, with the seven major chakras on the body forming a rainbow.

It takes much training in developing your intuition to correctly read an aura. The first seven chakras are the easiest to see. The last five are more difficult to perceive.

A distinct advantage of working with the color rays is their application to affected trouble areas. The infusion of radiant color balances, soothes, clears, and electrifies the weakened areas. However, as with any positive act, the effects last only as long as they are not overcome by negative, less-lighted actions or thoughts. If allowed to take hold, the person must then clear the negativity. There are several possible means: therapy or counseling, physical or cellular bodywork, mental and emotional clearing work,* or realignment of the spiritual body within the other three bodies (physical, mental, and emotional).

For these next several paragraphs, please refer to Chart 2-1.

The first three chakras (base, spleen, and solar plexus) are the **physical** chakras. They are directly connected to the physical body. We involve these when we wish to ground, or express ourselves in an earthy, sexual, or power-oriented way.

The heart chakra is the **transitional** chakra, the point between physical and non-physical. In other words, it is neither classified as a physical nor non-physical center; it is a link between the two. It is also an emotional chakra.

---

* See Chapter 10

An emotional chakra is directly connected to the emotional body.

The throat chakra is an emotional chakra which is part of the **non-physical** set of chakras. These non-physical chakras also include the third eye and the crown centers which are directly connected to our mental and spiritual bodies. A non-physical chakra carries a very strong spiritual energy that connects you to the subtle energies. The third eye and the crown are mental/spiritual chakras.

The chakras outside of the physical body (the eighth through the twelfth) are **etheric** chakras. The etheric chakras are pure, spiritual energy.[*] The silver and the gold chakras represent Love and Light respectively. The last three centers - white, clear, and black - form a triad of energy which is repeated throughout Creation. They represent free will and balance.

The Endocrine System and the Chakras

In medical science we have been able to document how specific physical functions perform. It is harder for us to prove the impact that the subtler chakra system has on our emotional and mental bodies, not to mention the physical body itself. The metaphysician sees the chakras as having a direct connection to the endocrine system (a system of ductless glands). The chakras also serve as a nerve network, tied to particular organs of the *physical* body.

The endocrine glands secrete hormones directly into the tissues and the capillary system (providing arterial/venous circulation to the cells of the body). They maintain a homeostatic environment, creating physical balance

---

[*] See Chapter 17

within the body by cooperating with the nervous system to facilitate the functions of reproductive activity, metabolic stability, and growth.

The endocrine/immune system can be directly linked to the seven major chakras (energy points) in the body. Each gland is associated with a particular chakra. When a chakra is out of alignment, or out of balance in its male/female energies, it eventually has a detrimental effect on the glandular system of the body. Likewise, when one of the glands weakens, it directly impacts the chakra system. Specifically, the immune system produces white blood cells that carry antibodies which protect the body against disease. The glandular system keeps the cells in balance through hormonal secretions. In short, our immune and glandular systems are our defense against illness and poor health.

The red **base** chakra (also called the first or the root chakra) corresponds with the gonads and ovaries. The kundalini energy (the Hindu word for "life force") coils upward from this chakra, and it is the chakra most connected to the earth. The testes and ovaries are, of course, integral parts of the reproductive cycle. Without them, it would be impossible to procreate.

The orange **spleen** center (also called the second or sexual chakra) is connected with the spleen and the pancreas. Creative energy and vitality are associated at this chakra. Insulin is secreted by the pancreas, affecting glucose levels in the body. The spleen filters the blood and is very active in the immune process; in fact, it is considered an organ of the immune system.

The yellow **solar plexus** chakra, or third chakra, is where the adrenal glands are connected. This is the primary point of power and emotions in the body. Epinephrine is released from these glands thereby stimulating the metabolic rate, the "fight or flight" reaction in life threatening situations. It is also involved with the breakdown of fatty acids and starches in the body.

The green/rose **heart** chakra (the fourth or transitional chakra) is linked to the thymus gland. This is the focal point of unconditional love and compassion. The thymus is a part of the lymph system; in fact, it plays a critical role in the protection of the immune system. Generally, as we age, the thymus ultimately atrophies. This is not something one needs to accept or "buy into". There are methods of keeping the thymus activated. One commonly used method is to briskly tap several times with the fingertips the sternum area over the thymus. Also, thymus vitamin supplements can be taken.

The translucent blue **throat** center, the fifth chakra, is associated with the thyroid gland. The throat is the seat of communication and self-expression in the body. The thyroid gland secretes a hormone, thyroxin, which increases oxygen consumption within the body, directly impacting the metabolic rate.

The indigo **third eye** chakra (also called the brow center, or sixth chakra) corresponds with the pituitary gland. Psychic and mental abilities are linked with this chakra. The pituitary gland's overactivity or underactivity is associated with growth and size of the body. It also directly stimulates the reproductory hormones.

The violet **crown** center (also called the seventh chakra or the *thousand-petal lotus*, an Eastern term describing an individual's ability to experience profound knowledge and direct wisdom of the Source) connects with the pineal gland. This is the seat of wisdom, unity, and liberation in the body. By opening and activating this chakra, one becomes in tune with God or the Source. The pineal's function is not clearly understood by the medical profession, but it is believed that it plays a role in the regulation of the sex glands, and the production of melatonin. Like the thymus gland, it also gradually degenerates. There is hope, however, for regenerating the pineal gland by using new ways that some ambitious researchers are studying, such as concepts aimed at halting the aging process. For example, transmitting color at the crown center helps to stabilize and strengthen the pineal gland.

The 13 Rays of Creation

My spiritual guides inform me that they see the universe as having 13 distinct rays that form the rainbow of energy that spirals out of the Source of Creation, or God. At this level, the 3rd dimension, the rays are perceived as pigments. As you climb up the dimensional levels, the colors become more radiant. The chakra system in the human body mirrors these divine rays exactly.

One comes into physical existence under the protective umbrella of one particular ray. Each of the 13 rays, or energies, represents a particular learning lesson. It appears that the Source set it up so that each ray exemplifies not only specific aptitudes of expression, but challenges and tests that expression. (See Chart 2-2)

Rays can be blended for use in healing. You will find, as you go along, that these blended rays start to automatically come through you.

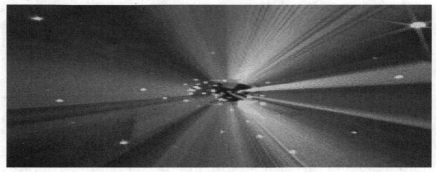

The Rays at the Physical Level

Red	The first of the physical colors. Warm. A good color for grounding your essence into the physical body. Wonderful for energizing a fatigued body.
Orange	A physical color. Warm. Good for creativity, vitality, and sexual expression.
Yellow	A physical color. Warm. Very good for getting in touch with your power. Deals with human ego and self-love.
Green	Physical healing. A blend of warm and cool. The all-purpose healer. ("When in doubt, use green")
Rose	Emotional healing. Warm Unconditional love energy.
Translucent Blue	Emotional. Cool. Excellent for communication.
Indigo	Mental/Spiritual. Cool. Excellent for clairvoyance and mental activity.
Violet	Spiritual. Cool. Wisdom. Enlightenment.
Silver	Feminine energy of Creation. The cosmic "Mother" energy. Use it to balance the female part of you.
Gold	Masculine energy of Creation. The cosmic "Father" energy. Use it to balance the male part of you.
White	Protection energy. Contains all the rays within it. Surround yourself in it to provide protection from dubious energy.
Clear	Truth and clarity. Contains all the rays within it. To achieve a clearer vision of Truth.
Black	Movement, grounding, and testing. Contains all the rays within it. Good for energy blockages, stagnation, and lack of good grounding. (See chapter 16 for more in-depth explanation.)

Chart 2-2

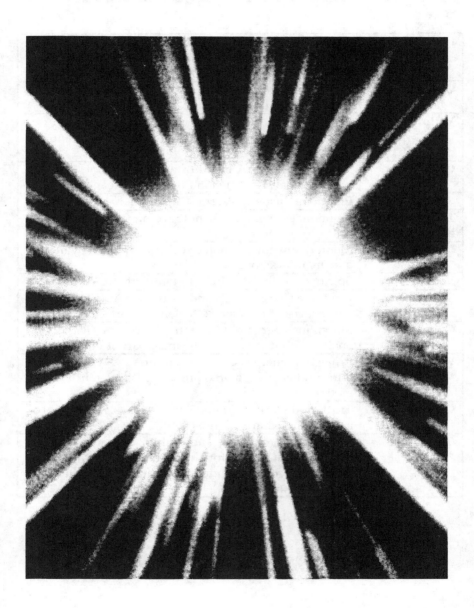

Chapter 3

The Basics

The Beginning

*From the Point of Light
within the center of Love*

*We move ever brighter
to become as one.*

*All are Light
All are Love.*

---Hatonn
8-26-91

Grounding, Balancing, Protection, and Clearing

There are several points I need to emphasize regarding the process of facilitating healing for others. Just as you would not want to scuba dive without the proper equipment, it would be ill-advised, even suicidal, not to follow some critical steps in the healing process. As harsh as it sounds, to wade into the energy stream of healing without knowing how to swim can be deadly. As you study and use the various techniques of energy transferal explained in this book, you'll see that there are several very important rules to follow. I call these *the basics*.

The four basics are **grounding**, **balancing**, **protection**, and **clearing**.

How to Ground

The first rule is **grounding**. The most effective healer is the one who is grounded in the 3rd dimension. Haven't you noticed how often people "have their lights on but nobody's home?" There are many reasons for this. Perhaps. the person is conflicted about being "present" or even being alive on Earth. I can't count the number of times I have heard people state that they wish they didn't have to be here; that living on Earth is too difficult, that humankind is too abusive and self-destructive. Arguably, the metaphysical bottom line is that you have *chosen* to be here (or you wouldn't be!), to function on this plane, perhaps in service to other beings. You have a responsibility to yourself as well. This includes embracing the 3rd dimensional experience in which you are residing. However, always be aware that you are a higher-dimensional

18

being, capable of accessing other planes of awareness. Remember that you "can be *in* the world, but not *of* it." The grounding process puts one in contact with Mother Earth as well as one's own body. Grounding honors both.

- One common method of grounding is to visualize a cord or tie from your tailbone going deep into the earth to secure it. It is best to see it anchored firmly inside the earth by a large crystal or stone. Remember, *thoughts are things* and by visualizing it you have literally created it in your energy field. An interesting and observable occurrence of this concept can be duplicated in this manner: A person is seated in a chair and visualizes a grounding cord tied from his tailbone into the earth. He mentally visualizes this but does not tell anyone. He creates the width and color of this cord. If another individual places her sensing hand under the chair where the cord is, she would be able to perceive a definite energy field approximating the diameter and color of the cord. She would either feel, see, hear, or know the nature of the cord.

Another method of grounding is to visualize specific colors. You may choose the green, gold, or black rays. One such technique is:

- Visualize the chosen color traveling up one of your feet, up that leg, then your hip, to the solar plexus chakra.
- Visualize it crossing over to the other side and down that hip, down the leg, and out the foot into the earth.
- Repeat for at least two more revolutions.

Note: *Do not bring the rays higher than the last physical chakra, which is the solar plexus. To ground involves only the physical energy and the physical chakras.*

Another variation of this technique is:

- Stand with your feet apart, arms at your sides with palms downward.
- Picture the gold ray traveling through your receptive hand, up the arm. Allow it to cross your solar plexus chakra and go down the other arm, out your transmitting hand into the earth.
- The gold ray mingles with the rich brown energy of Mother Earth and emerges as a tan-colored ray. Visualize it traveling up one leg, across the solar plexus chakra once more, then down the other leg back into the earth.
- Do this last step one more time.

Here's one more good grounding technique:

Grounding Your Higher Self into Your Physical Body

- Stand with your feet slightly apart with your hands by your side. Visualize a silver ray containing ruby red coming from the earth into your hands.
- Inhale deeply as you move your hands above your head. Exhale as you place your hands back by your side. Repeat three times.
- Visualize the green ray coming from the earth into the bottoms of your feet. Allow this ray to travel the complete length of your body and exit at the crown. Repeat three times.
- Place the right hand above the crown chakra with the palm of the hand facing your body. Touch each chakra with the middle finger of the right hand with the intent of closing them at the *emotional* body level. Repeat this three times.
- Place the left hand above the crown chakra with the palm of the hand facing your body. Touch each chakra with the middle finger of the right hand with the in-

tent of closing them at the *physical* body level. Repeat three times.
- Place both hands together and touch the crown chakra, the heart chakra, and the base chakra. Repeat three times.

How to Balance

The second discipline is **balance**. This is probably the hardest point to practice and the hardest to maintain. To be in balance, ideally, is to have no blocks in your physical, emotional, and mental bodies. It also means that your spiritual body is aligned with the rest of you. Perfect balance is seldom seen. If we were perfect beings we would not, necessarily, even be here on Earth. We can be diligent people and respect ourselves by becoming ever more balanced daily. It is then that we will be able to help ourselves and others as we progress along life's journey of self-discovery and self-transformation.

"To bring into proportion or harmony" is the way Webster's Dictionary defines balance. This definition can be applied to financial books of a corporation, the grandeur of the forces of nature, to animals, and to human beings.

What really makes up a human being?

A human being is a complex individual who has physical, emotional, and mental bodies with his soul as the nucleus of his essence.

In other words, man and woman are composed of several *bodies*, or *aspects*, with the soul as the key component expressing through their various bodies.

Most often we see individuals who predominately express themselves through one aspect of their being, frequently ignoring, or giving little thought to, the others. For example, a man may have very good mental characteristics but completely denies the emotional part of his being. Frequently, we see women who are quite emotional but do not use their logical mind as often. Or just the opposite; a woman who has used her logical mind all her life, but has no idea how to express herself emotionally... or a man who accepts his emotions but doesn't give much attention to his logical mind.

Then there are the extremes of expression. For example: the person who has an imbalance in his or her emotional state, may frequently give vent to non-productive expressions of emotion such as jealousy, rage, repressed anger, and the like.

Here is one that those in the metaphysical realms may recognize: the person who spends most of his life detached from the body, then wonders why his body is very unhappy with that state of affairs and is sick or otherwise out-of-balance. There is nothing wrong with the conscious, spiritual practice of the out-of-body state, but you must give the body its due by loving, supporting, and accepting its role in your life. The other extreme is the totally physically involved individual who cannot connect with his spiritual side.

So, why be in balance? What do we get from it? Those people who live a balanced existence find greater happiness and well-being. They have a fuller self-expression since they do not have the blocks.

What does it mean to be truly in balance?

Being in balance allows the flow of Love and Light to be transmitted through your essence without blockages.

Without such blockages, the Love and Light (like water traveling through an unkinked pipe) are not restricted in their flow through any of the bodies; physical, mental, or emotional, and the spiritual body becomes aligned within those bodies. This gives rise to full expression of your gifts and abilities.

How do we get our body, mind, and emotions in balance?

1. Spiritually, by:
    *   Allowing the universal flow of Light and Love to manifest in your life,
    *   Continuously tuning into, and opening up to this flow,
    *   Knowing what role you play in this great Cosmic Drama,
    *   Realizing that your role, no matter how small, is an integral part of the drama. Without you, it would not be the same. At a spiritual level, each of us has formulated a blueprint or **intent** for our lifetime. It is impressed onto our souls, and hopefully utilized and expressed by each of our bodies. Often we consciously forget what our intent is.
2. Mentally, by:
    *   Allowing the universal flow of Light and Love to manifest by *clarifying* through **data** your game plan or spiritual intent,
    *   Clearing all unnecessary mental debris blocking the original pure spiritual intent.

3. Clearing away the emotional debris allows your emotional **expression** to reflect the pure spiritual intent and correct mental data.

4. And finally, physically clearing the cellular, physical body allows the physical **manifestation** of the spiritual intent, balanced mental data, and emotional expression. Voila! You are in balance. (See Chapter 10 on the clearing processes for a more detailed explanation.)

Many of us are not extremely out of balance. We have our moments of clarity and well-being. We just seem to find it difficult to maintain a state of balance continuously. As we continue to develop our talents, nurture and align all our bodies, use the checks and balances of spiritual intent, mental data, emotional expression, and physical manifestation--we will achieve that balance.

The following technique is an excellent exercise for balancing the physical, emotional, and mental bodies, while aligning the spiritual body into the other three:

LaLur's Balancing Technique

1) Stand with your feet slightly apart and palms down at the level of your solar plexus. (Fig. 3.1a)
2) Visualize the *gold* ray coming into the crown chakra and flowing through your body. (See Chart 2-1 for the chakra locations.)
3) Allow the ray to exit your transmitting hand and enter into the earth. As the ray flows through the earth, it will begin to pick up the color of the planet, the wonderful brown richness found there.
4) This ray will then flow upward into the receiving hand across the solar plexus through the transmitting arm, then back into the earth. (Repeat this three times and on the third time allow the ray to remain in the earth.)
5) Move your hands to the level of your heart chakra. Bring forth the *emerald green* ray of healing into the

crown chakra through your body to the transmitting hand and down into the earth. (Fig. 3.1b)

6) Allow the ray to flow up to your receiving hand across your heart chakra and exit out your transmitting hand back into the earth. (Repeat three times.)

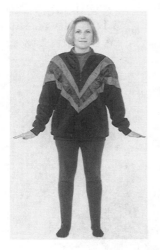 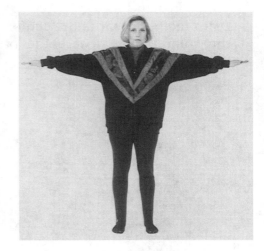

Fig 3.1a   Fig 3.1b

7) Raise your hands above your head, palms up. Bring forth the *violet* ray into your crown chakra. Allow the ray to flow down your body through the receiving side and up your body to exit via your transmitting hand into the ethers. (Repeat three times.) (Fig. 3.1c)

8) Follow these hand movements to close the three levels of the chakras. (These are movements from the healing orders of the other levels):

9) With arms still overhead during Step 7, bring down your left hand along the center line of your body, your palm facing towards the center. (Fig. 3.1d) Go as far as the solar plexus where the palm is switched towards the left side.

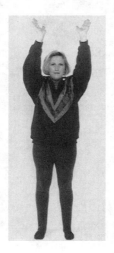
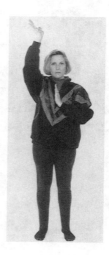

Fig 3.1c   Fig 3.1d

10) Bring down your other hand, palm facing towards the center. (Fig. 3.1e) Go as far as the heart chakra where your palm is switched towards the right side.
11) Bring your palms together at the heart chakra in a prayer-like position. (Fig. 3.1f)

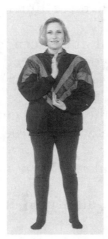

Fig 3.1e

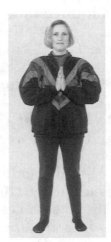

Fig 3.1f

Male/Female Balancing

Your chakras should be equally balanced in the masculine and feminine energies, whether you are a male or a female. The purpose of this exercise is to balance the male and female energies at each of the chakras. Initially, become proficient at rotating the chakras three times in each direction. This exercise involves balancing the physical body.

- Visualize your red *base* chakra as a disk, turning three times to the left, then three times to the right. Rotate it gently, but firmly.

  Note: If there is difficulty in turning any of your chakras either direction, it shows imbalance in the male or female energy. Counter-clockwise direction is female, clockwise is male.

- Next, go to the orange *spleen* chakra, seeing it as a disk and turning it three times to the left, then three times to the right.
- Travel psychically to the yellow *solar plexus* chakra. Turn it three times to the left, then three times to the right.
- At the *heart* chakra you can turn the green chakra first, then do the rose chakra, or you can blend them like a watermelon tourmaline (a pink and green gem).
- Go to the *throat* chakra and see the translucent blue disk. Turn it three times to the left, then three times to the right.
- Next, see the indigo *third eye* chakra. Turn it three times to the left, three to the right.
- Finally, the violet *crown* chakra disk--turn it three times in both directions.

As you become proficient at turning the chakras, you may increase the turns clockwise and counter-clockwise to seven times each. Eventually you can increase the number of rotations to thirteen times each direction. Seven times involves balancing the physical, emotional, and mental bodies. Thirteen involves balancing the physical, emotional, and mental aspects, while aligning the spiritual body.

You can learn to perceive the chakras of others and discern how they are flowing. As you become more attuned to sensing, you can either feel, know, or see the spinning of each chakra using your receiving or sensing hand.

How to Spiritually Protect Yourself

The next point is **protection**. This simply means that you have a say in the type of energies that come through you in the healing mode, and the type of non-physical beings you wish to surround yourself with on a regular basis. Specifically, on this point of protection, I am referring to the energies that you bring forth in the channeling process. Unfortunately, not all non-physical energies are benevolent. Some wish to manipulate and control. Protection gives you the armor with which to insulate yourself from such beings. Do you prefer an evolved, symbiotic essence to communicate with you or one who wishes to control? You make that choice. If you are open to the channeling process, you are wide open. That is why you must be selective about what you will allow through you.

Protection means "the act of shielding oneself from physical, emotional, mental, or spiritual injury." By calling forth the Light and Love of Creation, God or the Source, you automatically set up the conditions of protection already built in. Chinks in the armor of that protection result from the "four deadly sins" of ego, greed, adultery, and fear, along with a severe lack of boundaries.

Ego, greed, and fear are fairly self-explanatory, but adultery has a somewhat different meaning than you may think. To commit adultery (in my spiritual guides' definition), means to attempt to alter someone to fit your expectations. This definition is actually close to the word *adulterate*, or to make impure by changing the substance of something. The common biblical definition is to have sexual intercourse with someone else's spouse, but this is not how the word is being used here.

As was stated previously, by invoking the "Light of the Source or God," you set the proper vibrational conditions and energies for healing. I have used a little prayer for years which originally came from the Unity Church:

"The Light of God surrounds me,
The Love of God enfolds me,
The Power of God protects me,
The Presence of God watches over me.
Wherever I am, God is.
So be it."

Another excellent method of protection is to invoke the *white* ray of light which specifically protects, and the *clear* ray that represents discernment and truth at all levels. By asking for these rays with a positive intent you will attract them to you. They will set up a strong protective barrier around your essence.

Another effective exercise in alignment and protection goes as follows:

Affirmation, Alignment and Protection

Personally, I acknowledge, I bless, I align, all parts of me
I am yesterday, I am today, I am tomorrow
I call forth the angels of the four corners-
Michael [North-Fire]
Gabriel [South-Earth]
Ariel   [East -Air]
Uriel   [West -Water]
To set the four corners within this place*.
I invoke the White Brotherhood† symbol
to cloak all in protection.

---

* You may specify workplace, home, car, hotel room, etc.

† A non-physical, spiritual order of ascended masters. Their symbol is a magenta color circle containing a white cross.

*I go forth this day in Light and Love,
with Free Will and Balance*,
knowing who I am and what I represent.*

How to Clear

The last point to emphasize is **clearing**. Think of yourself as a magnet that can attract or repel energy. Your aura **is** magnetic. Too much of the time it carries within it *other people's stuff* ! In other words, you pick up the vibrations of others, whether positive or negative in nature. When you come into contact with fellow beings, you exchange auric energy. You often get more than you bargained for. Now I am not saying that you should become a hermit so you can keep your aura "pure." Just become aware of what is yours and what isn't. Your own issues offer you more than enough to deal with.

My spiritual teachers have given me a wonderful technique for clearing. I visualize a shower oi multi-colored light pouring over me, resembling a shower of water. By mentally invoking this image, we **will** create it. Through our intuitive sight we are able to see the multi-colored rainbow flood through the aura, clearing away all debris.

A good physical method of clearing is to immerse yourself for at least 15 minutes in a warm bath with a cup or two of Epsom salts. Epsom salt is an excellent auric clearer, but its real claim to fame is as a cellular, emotional, and mental body cleanser.

If you are clearing your energy between clients, or are not near a tub for a full bath, you can immerse your hands

---

* The four universal laws of creation

in Epsom salts to transmute the excess energy. Two or three minutes should be adequate.

A cup or two of apple cider vinegar is a very good toxin cleanser. Placed in the bath water, we have found it effective in clearing malathion, chlorine, metals, chemicals, etc., from the tissues of the body. I have malathion and chlorine sensitivities; it is the only method I have found that can eliminate them from my system.

Another way of cleansing the aura is the use of 4-8 ounces of baking soda in the bath. It brightens the aura; it also helps to clear the effects of having had X-rays.

Clearing Excess or Unwanted Energy

- Dip your hands in cool water, feeling the excess or unwanted energy being transmuted (altered into another form of energy).

or

- Perform a wiping motion of the hands, feeling the unnecessary energy being sloughed off.

or

- Say "All that is not mine let drop away from me NOW."

To release excess energy and help keep your ego out of the way, do the following invocation:

"I invoke the Light/Energy of Source to run through me.
I allow myself to be a clear and perfect channel.
I don't own the energy.
I don't hold the energy.
I simply move the energy."

Ways to Keep Your Chakra System in Alignment

- Do male/female balancing, grounding, clearing, and protection work every day
- Allow the clearing process to proceed at a rate that is not too uncomfortable (See Chapter 10)
- Frequent Epsom salt and apple cider vinegar baths
- Be willing to look at your issues, get counseling or other support if you need it
- Have frequent body work; e.g. chiropractic, acupuncture, massage therapy, color energy therapy, etc.
- Maintain a good daily diet and vitamin therapy. Specific supplements may be needed (such as thyroid or adrenal) to boost your immunity
- Healthful and sufficient exercise for the body; e.g. walking, swimming, aerobics, etc.
- Practice regular meditation and other spiritual forms of expression to align all four of your bodies; e.g. light or sound therapies, Tai Chi, channeling, etc.

Preparation for Dealing With Psychic Energy

Frequently, when you get involved in psychic or healing work, you have to deal with new levels and quantities of energy that your body is not accustomed to. You have a large capacity for Source energy to run through you, though it may sometimes feel like having 220 volts of energy going through a 110 volt body.

The following are techniques that have worked for my students. There is no one method that works for everyone. After awhile, you may find that you can eliminate one or more of these suggestions, except the dietary suggestions, Epsom salt baths, and drinking sufficient quantities of water.

1. Eat enough protein such as nuts and leafy green vegetables. Eat minimal amounts of sugar, or none at all. Cheese is acceptable only if your body can tolerate it.
2. Check your tolerance for wearing metals or crystals during the healing process. (This is mainly a concern for those who are extra sensitive and may not be able to take the amplified, stored energy that the crystals and metals retain.)
3. Drink water frequently (with lemon added is good) during the course of the healing session.
4. Look for electronic devices in the healing area. Some, such as sonic flea elimination instruments, can disturb the electromagnetic field of the body.
5. Initially, have a trained healer be a facilitator for you, monitoring for such things as groundedness, clearing, etc..
6. As mentioned previously, Epsom salts may be used to ground your body and balance the energy after the experience. Apply it to your hands; if you are able to take a bath, do so.
7. In the rare instance that there is evidence of *psychic shock*, take Bach Flower "Rescue Remedy™." * Signs of psychic shock include: shakiness or dizziness, skin looks pale or feels clammy, tears, inability to ground.

---

* Four flower essences that specifically calm the emotional body. A concoction of one or two tablespoons of blackstrap molasses and the juice of half a lemon in warm water can be substituted for "Rescue Remedy."

8. Use dried sage and cedar to smudge* the physical space you've been working in. It clears the area of unwanted energies. You will definitely feel a lighter, clearer energy.
9. Another way to clear your auric field is to surround yourself in aromatherapy[†], either by applying it directly to the body or by the use of a diffuser unit that disperses the essential oil throughout your work space.

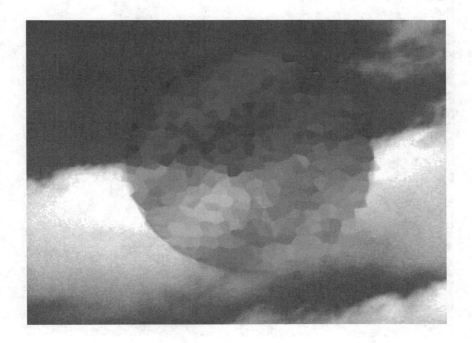

---

* To "smudge", a Native American tradition, place dried sage and cedar (available at health food or New Age stores) in a pottery bowl. Light a flame, then snuff it out, producing ample smoke. Allow the smoke to permeate the physical space and your auric field.

[†] The ancient art of using scent as a healing tool

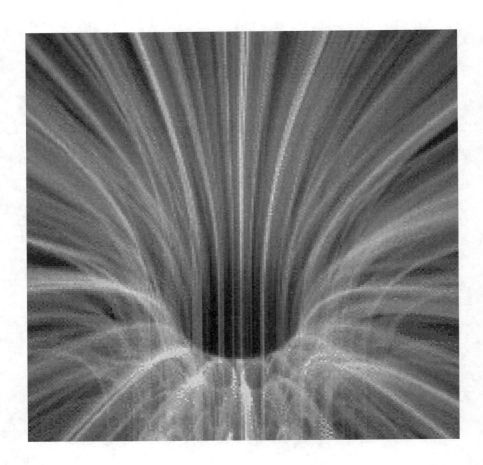

Chapter 4

Channeling the Energy

═══════════════════════

I Am

I am a vessel
I am a tool

I am a passage
for Light to move

I am connection
I am the mass

I am the channel
for Love to pass

---Alana
July 1991

The word "channeling" is very popular in the New Age lingo; perhaps, it is even overused. But few words really express the process of allowing yourself to be a vehicle, a conduit for the flow of universal Love and Light. *It is who and what we are.* The process benefits those entities who allow interaction with us; it also helps ourselves and our own alignment and empowerment. Usually it's not difficult to open the channel; the hard part is monitoring the energy and turning it down on command.

Once you commit to working with the Light, you change your life irrevocably. You are no longer the same person you were. You become the person you were meant to be.

The first step in channeling energy is to ascertain in what manner you naturally run and sense the energy. In order to do this you must determine which hand transmits energy and which receives.

Determining your Transmitting Hand

- Place your arms comfortably in your lap, palms upward, fingers uncurled.
- Have another person place his or her own hands, palms downward about six inches above your palms, not touching physically.
- Ask the person to feel the energy emanating from your palms. Ask him or her to determine which one emanates more energy. This is your transmitting hand because more energy is flowing outward.
- If the energy emanating is equal from both palms, then both your hands are capable of transmitting. This is called being *ambidextrous.*

- If the energy is almost equal, you have the capability of being ambidextrous if you practice "running the energy," and focus on using both hands to transmit.

Determining Your Sensing Hand

- Place your arms comfortably in your lap, palms upward, fingers uncurled.
- Have another person place his or her own hands, palms downward about six inches above your palms, not touching physically.
- Ask the person to feel the energy emanating from your palms. Ask him or her to determine which one emanates less energy. This is your sensing or receiving hand because less energy is flowing outward.
- If the energy emanating is equal from both palms, then both your hands are capable of sensing. This is called being *ambidextrous*.
- If the energy is almost equal, you have the capability of being ambidextrous if you practice "sensing the energy," and focus on using both hands to sense.

The Crystallization Process

Since color therapy involves the healing touch of your hands, you can amplify your effectiveness by using techniques that will increase the amount of energy that flows through the palms of your hands. The following technique involves placing an "amplifying" crystal in each palm chakra of the subtle energy *body*:

- Close your eyes. Still your wayward thoughts as you assume a meditative position. Feel yourself beginning to tune into your Divine essence--to Life itself. *This is your true nature.*
- Visualize the flow of that Essence entering your crown chakra, flowing down your spine to your arms. It is a rainbow of pastel colors--hues and shades unknown on this dimension because of their pure state.
- Feel the energy increase in the top of your head. Feel the sensation of warmth as the energy builds. Allow the rainbow of colors to gently flood into your being.
- Now look at the palms of your hands. Imagine the gathered energy turning into crystalline form. Visualize the solidified crystals as they turn emerald green in color. They pulsate with a pure, unearthly emerald green light.
- Know that you now have an amplified energy that you may call on when needed. Only use it for the highest good.
- Now release the energy; send it to those in need of healing. Ground yourself.

Opening Up to Your Guidance

Everyone on Earth has a number of spiritual guides and guardians to give counsel, protect, inspire, and generally help them. These spiritual guides would be considered etheric or nonphysical, at least not physical as we know it. They may reside at any level or dimension, from the 4th through the 12th planes. (For an in-depth discussion of the different dimensions, see Chapter 17.) These guides are willing and able to give guidance, though we usually ignore those subtle hints or feelings, even passing them off as imagination or dreaming.

The purpose of the following meditation is to help you meet one of your guides, someone who will help you with your channeling of multidimensional energy. This exercise will also better attune you to the inner dimensions:

- Center your essence. Feel the God-self within; your individualized soul connected to the Source. Feel that Oneness.
- Now ask for the rainbow rays of Light to ignite your consciousness. The multi-hued and multi-faceted spectrum of light energy will flow in a spiral motion.
- Observe the colors with your inner sight as they manifest within and around you. (If you can't see the colors, don't worry. Many do not see them, at first. Pretend or imagine that you see them. This is called *visualization*.)
- Feel how light your body is because you are no longer sensing the denseness of the physical body. Your essence is being temporarily freed from that density. Let it soar upward--free! *You and the Light are One.*
- Now allow the rainbow rays of Light to take you to a faraway place, a deeper understanding of a new level of consciousness; an inner dimension of mind.
- Next, ask your spiritual guides to give you some sort of symbol that will have meaning for you, a symbol that will instantly attune you to the inner planes and your ever present guides.
- After you perceive a symbol, bid "good-bye" to your guides. Thank them for their help. Allow the rainbow rays of Light to bring you back to your physical body.
- Ground yourself carefully.

You may visualize and connect with your symbol whenever you want to tune into divine guidance from your inner self.

Color Visualization Technique

The art of creative visualization is a powerful tool for manifesting whatever you desire in life. It brings your spiritual intent forth and grounds it into your physical reality. It utilizes your physical visual sight and your internal psychic sight. It is multidimensional and what we term *holographic,* the process which integrates and aligns all aspects of yourself.

- Sit or lie comfortably. Set the energy of protection around you by invoking either the angels of the four corners (Michael, Gabriel, Ariel, and Uriel), or by asking for the protective energy of the Source of All.
- Notice any tense areas in your body. Gently tighten that area of tension, then release it. Feel the tension leaving. Do this with each taut area in the body.
- Breathe deeply and evenly, feeling the cleansing power of oxygen permeating your body's cells as you inhale, and the release of carbon dioxide waste as you exhale. Conscious, deep breathing honors the physical, emotional, and mental bodies by facilitating the unblocking of the life force while embracing the beauty of your physical expression. This allows your spiritual Higher Self to align in the body.
- Visualize the crown chakra (at the top of your head) begin to open as though it were the lens of a camera. Ask for all 13 rays of rainbow energy to flow down through your crown. These rainbow colors are the red, orange, yellow, green, rose, translucent blue, indigo,

violet, silver, gold, white, clear, and black rays. They are present at all 13 dimensional levels, and can be pulled from whichever level is appropriate for you at this time. By stating this intent they will flow from the right dimension for your use. Do not be concerned if you don't know about each dimension; by asking for the right one(s), it will happen.

- As the rainbow rays flow into your crown chakra, see them enter your bloodstream through the arteries, arterioles, capillaries, and veins. Watch them flow through all the neurons (nerve cells) and synapses (nerve cell connections) throughout the brain area. There are estimated to be between 10 and 100 billion neurons in your body. Most of these are in your brain. The brain is not only responsible for all sensory input and motor activities. It also oversees involuntary functions such as breathing, heart rate, and blood pressure. Our precious brains supervise all the creative endeavors, as well as logical thinking and emotions.

  To take it a step further, the brain is the seat of psychic perception and abilities; processes we as a people have ignored for many centuries. These dormant psychic processes can be awakened by the application of the 13 rays of light energy.

- At this time, see the "rainbow blood" move through what my guides call the *tensor* center of the brain, the psychic center of perception. This tensor center is located in the middle of the brain. With intensity of thought, focus the rainbow colored blood through your tensor area. This part of your brain will gradually awaken when this exercise is regularly practiced.

- Next, allow the rainbow blood to flow down the neck, shoulders, arms, torso, legs, and feet. See this rainbow energy coursing along through your blood vessels, just as your own blood is pumped through the body.

Your blood consists of red cells, white cells, platelets, and plasma. Your red cells carry oxygen to all other body cells, your white cells fight disease, and the platelets stop deadly leaks through the clotting process. Your plasma, which is mostly water, carries the blood cells, platelets, nutrients, and hormones. Feel the rainbow blood electrify your physical blood, rebalancing any imbalance.

- As the rainbow blood travels through each portion of your body, feel it revitalize any weakened areas, and enhance any normal areas.
- Keep the rainbow blood coursing through your body as long as you can comfortably visualize it. Just keep it circulating from your head to your feet and back again.
- To bring the technique to an end, just allow the rays to dissipate, clearing the excess energy from your auric field by sending the energy down into the earth. Your spiritual intent will be for the planet to use it for clearing, healing, and aligning.
- Close your crown chakra to a comfortable, normal position.
- Ground yourself to the earth.

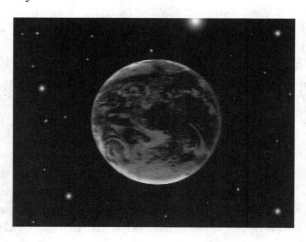

Chapter 5
Energy Reading and Body Scanning

Who am I

Thousands of Spectrums
Lights ever moving.

Energy waves electric
Signatures, signs of essence.

---Mira
8-26-91

Seeing or Sensing Energy

Energy reading is really in the eye of the beholder. It is not an exact science, but one of subjective perception. Each energy reader will bring his or her own interpretations of what the colors mean, and how the *auric* picture as a whole tells a story. Does this mean one will never get an accurate or complete picture? Not at all. What it means is this: If you had a group of ten skilled energy readers give their impressions of one person, you would most likely get ten slices of the whole pie, each slice would contain some part of the truth. One reader may sense that the person is a creative storyteller, another may "pick up" his empathy, another his math ability. One reader may perceive exactly the same thing as another reader. All the traits of the person may be accurate, and combined they give us a picture of the person's nature.

Psychic perception is obtained in one of four ways:
1. Seeing (visual or clairvoyant)
2. Feeling (empathic or clairsentience)
3. Hearing (auditory or clairaudience)
4. Knowing (wisdom or perception)

Clairvoyance is *visual* psychic ability as sensed through "psychic sight", energy, non-physical beings, and general psychic phenomena.

Clairsentience means *feeling* psychic ability as sensed through "psychic touch", energy, non-physical beings, and general psychic phenomena.

Clairaudience means *hearing* psychic ability as sensed through "psychic listening", energy, non-physical beings, and general psychic phenomena.

"Knowing" is *perceiving* cosmic wisdom by tuning into your inner self, energy, non-physical beings, and general psychic phenomena.

Normally, one of these psychic perceptions will appear to be your strongest ability, with the others available in varying strengths. The majority of healers seem to be strongest in clairsentience, but there are exceptions.

Eventually, when your energy blocks are gone, your clearing processes are complete (see Chapter 10), and you spend the majority of your time in alignment, all forms of psychic abilities will become your own.

Creating an energy ball is an excellent way to learn to feel or sense energy.

- With your arms parallel to the floor, and elbows bent, place your hands about a foot apart with the palms facing each other. Your fingers should be slightly bent. At first, you may wish to close your eyes to eliminate any visual distractions.
- Slowly bring your hands toward each other until you feel a sensation of either heat, tingling, or some other subtle difference. You have now encountered your energy field. It's that easy! When you have reached this point, stop moving your hands toward each other.
- Now lightly pat this energy field by moving the hands an inch closer to each other, then drawing them apart an inch or two. Feel as though you are holding a ball between your hands. As you do this, the sensation you are feeling will increase in intensity.
- When you are done experiencing your energy ball, drop your hands to your sides and think of sending the excess energy into the earth.

Here is a good method for seeing auras:
- Have a friend stand up against a white wall or door.
- Close your eyes halfway and allow yourself to achieve an alpha or meditative state of mind. Feel as relaxed as possible; tension makes it harder to tune in.
- You may begin to see colors against the white backdrop. Note what you are seeing so that you can describe it later. Notice also which colors appear near particular parts of the body. You will not necessarily *see* visually but will either *feel, hear,* or *know* which colors are in the aura.

A variation of this technique is to seat a person against a white sheet backdrop with a dim blue light behind it. Lower the lights.

Opening the Aura

Opening the aura means to penetrate another's electromagnetic field with healing energy (with their agreement). Sometimes, there may be fear-based resistance to the process. If that is the case, the aura may be as impenetrable as a brick wall. Healing energies will merely bounce off the aura without effect. When the other person gives you permission, that agreement allows the healing energies to permeate the auric field. The following is an exercise in opening an aura:
- Ask the person if he or she wants a healing. The consent given should be spoken aloud. (This shows a definite intent and willingness to receive a healing.)
- Place your hand at the crown chakra and the other hand at the forehead (third eye). (Fig. 5.1)

- Wait until you feel a warm sensation at the crown, which signifies that it is now open.
- If you do not feel a positive response, ask the person if he or she really desires the healing experience. They may opt for not having one at this time.

Closing an Aura

When you have completed a healing session, you will need to seal the aura. Do not leave the person wide open. It is too easy for undesirable energies to then pervade their auric field.

- Touch the crown chakra and simply state, "I am sealing your aura." (Fig. 5.2)

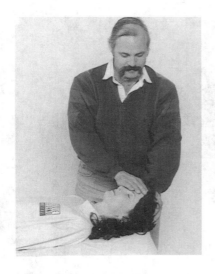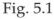
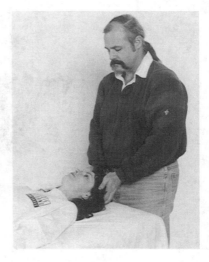

Fig. 5.1   Fig. 5.2

Body Scan Technique

The purpose of this exercise is to detect areas of imbalance within an auric field.

- Find a partner. Sit facing one another. Feel the aura by starting at the top of the head, with hands out at auric level. (Fig. 5.3)
- Areas with a disturbance will usually feel very hot or very cold. This may be either of a physical, emotional, or mental origin.
- When reaching a problem area, share with your partner your findings in order to determine if the issue is being held by the physical, emotional, or mental body or bodies.
- You may then send one or more specific color rays to the problem area(s).

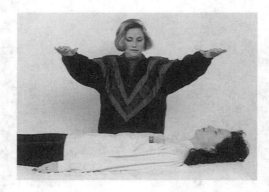

Fig. 5.3

Sending and Receiving Colors

Here is a technique I have used to specifically attune my students to the practice of sending and receiving colors:
- Work in pairs. Determine who will be receiving and who will be sending.
- The sender sits with elbows bent and the palms of both hands facing the receiver. He or she should choose a color and send it without telling the other person, allowing him or her to guess it.
- Another variation is to tell the other person the color prior to sending it. (This would probably be the best course for a beginner who is not accustomed to recognizing the rays.)
- If you are the receiver, simply allow yourself to be passive and open. When the color is sent, just see how it feels, or if you are particularly visual, see if you sense it.

If you don't have a partner, you can practice this alone. Simply allow the chosen color to flow through you, sending it out into the earth, or into your pet or plants. Feel or otherwise intuitively sense it. Practice receiving colors by subtly scanning your environment, and by noticing the auric fields around plants and animals.

Preparing for a Healing

The purpose of this exercise is to help you to attune with your guides prior to doing a healing session. After a while, you may find that it is no longer necessary to prepare in this manner; that the information flows to you without any major effort.

- Ask for the *lavender* light of wisdom, and the *emerald* ray of healing, to come through your crown chakra.
- Imagine the rays slowly passing through your face and head to fill your brain--touching each synaptical connection within the brain.
- Feel them flow down your neck and arms, then down your torso, hips, legs, ankles, and feet. Allow the rays to flow out the bottom of your feet.
- Before each healing, tune into your inner guidance. Feel the lavender and the emerald rays flow into your being. This will center all of your chakras. The rays will allow you to retrieve intuitive information regarding the person receiving your channeled healing.

Polarities of Male and Female Bodies

Each side of the human body has a negative or positive charge, electrically speaking. *Positive* means male, and *negative* means female, whether it is in the male or female body.

For males, the left side of their physical body is positive, and the right side is negative. For females, the left side of their physical body is negative, and the right side is positive.

A good way to remember this is that the brain is divided into two hemispheres--the right brain (creative, intuitive) and the left brain (logic). Think of the left brain as *male* and the right brain as *female*.

In the female, the *female* energy crosses diagonally to the left side of the body; the *male* energy crosses diagonally to the right side of the body. In the male, the *female* energy stays on the same side--the right; the *male* energy stays on the same side--the left. Only in the center of the body where the chakras are located is it the same for both male and female. This is the point of androgyny in the physical body. (See Chapter 6 -- Chakra Balancing)

When you are in a male (or positive) physical body, you have a feminine (or negative) emotional body, and a masculine (or positive) mental body. Conversely, when you are in a female (or negative) physical body, you have a masculine (or positive) emotional body, and a feminine (or negative) mental body. Of course, the soul energy is androgynous for both male and female physical bodies.

Knowing the positive (male) and negative (female) sides gives you valuable body scan information about those you are working with. You will be able to determine whether they have issues regarding their feminine or masculine nature, and/or issues with the males and females in their lives. You'll know if they are resistant to their logical or intuitive selves.

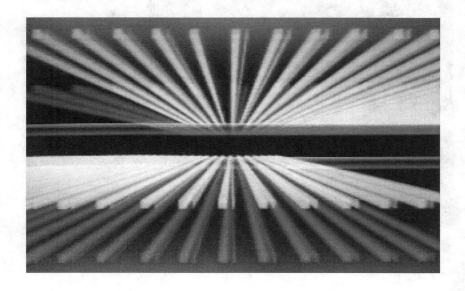

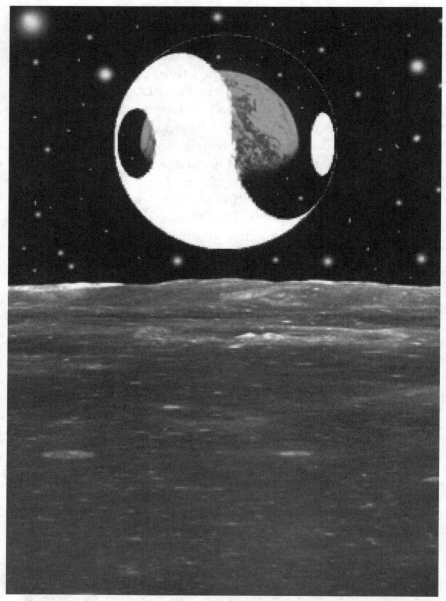

Sarah Steinbach

Chapter 6

Chakra Balancing

Yin/Yang

I am male
movement eternal

I am female
nurturing maternal

I am androgyny
I move, I nurture

I am maternal
I am eternal.

—Alana
8-26-91

Before performing the following technique of chakra balancing, you may wish to practice sensing another's chakras. Place your sensing hand over each chakra, noting two key points:

1. **Which way is the energy flowing?** The chakra will tend to have a natural pattern, flowing generally in one direction. That direction indicates an emphasis on either the male or female. Counter-clockwise rotation is female, clockwise rotation is male.

2. **Which chakras are not in balance?** The chakras where all of the energy movement flows one way, or where erratic movement is found, indicate imbalances. These discrepancies point to blocks, strengths, and weaknesses. For example, a female's second chakra that turns clockwise only, shows an imbalance in her female sexual energy. Erratic movement in a male's solar plexus chakra indicates issues with his empowerment and self-love. Perhaps, his self-expression is blocked; he might be upset over recent ego issues in his life, or any number of other issues. It is up to you, the color therapist, to facilitate his connection to the problem area and its implications. This can be done by pertinent intuitive questioning, or you can simply trigger an emotional reaction in him by applying energy to that point.

Chakra Balancing For Other People

You are now aware of the importance of keeping your own chakra system in balance. This chakra balancing technique will help your client, and hopefully show him or her the benefits attained by having balanced energy centers.

- Open the aura by receiving the person's consent for the healing.
- Place your three middle fingers of one hand at the base chakra in a triangle formation; place the three middle fingers of the other hand at the third eye, also in a triangle position. (Fig. 6.1)
- Leave your fingers in place until you intuitively feel the energies have been aligned (usually 2-3 minutes). You will either feel a diminishment of the energy flow, indicating completion, or perhaps *hear* the words, "It is complete."
- When you're finished, you may begin any other healing technique at this time. It is a good time to do a body scan, checking for troubled or imbalanced areas.
- Be prepared to discuss with your client what he or she may have experienced or felt.

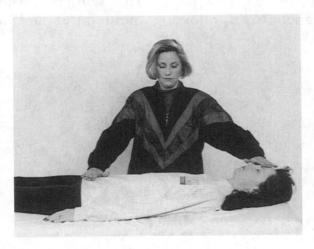

Fig. 6.1

Energy Transferal

The purpose of this technique is to help someone amplify his or her development in all four bodies. It cleans up negative or stale energies and infuses positive, uplifting spiritual energies. It is to be used on those who are spiritually ready to make a leap in consciousness.

Think of this technique as being similar to a carpet cleaning machine. It shoots water out of the hose into the carpet; at the same time it sucks in the dirty carpet water through the other part of the hose. The energy transferal technique transfers energy into the person at the same time it removes stagnant, inharmonious energy.

This exercise is to be done once a week, generally over a period of five weeks:

1) Have the person lie down on his/her back.
2) For 2 or 3 minutes, rotate your hands over the auric level of the person's body.* This will stir up the electromagnetic field, allowing more input and shifting. (Fig. 6.2a)

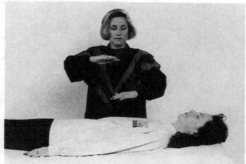

Fig. 6.2a

---

* This will impact the *energy meridians* (polarity map of the energy body). For the purposes of this exercise, it is not necessary to be aware of each individual energy meridian.

3) Place your hands on your client's shoulders as you channel healing energy into their body. (Fig. 6.2b)
4) Move your hands slowly, lightly but firmly, down the client's body from shoulders to toes.
5) Transmute excess or unwanted energy by rubbing your hands briskly together, or dipping them in water. (Fig. 6.2c)
6) Do the last two steps sequentially 7 times.
7) Now, repeat the process as you move down both arms, 7 times. Transmute the energy between each movement.

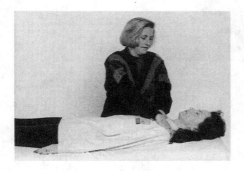

Fig. 6.2b

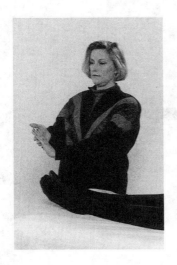

Fig. 6.2c

8) Have the person turn onto his/her stomach. Do the hand rotation, as described above in step 2, (Fig. 6.2d) followed by the "energy pulling and inputting" (as described above) down the body. (Fig. 6.2e) Do this 5 times with energy transmutation in between.

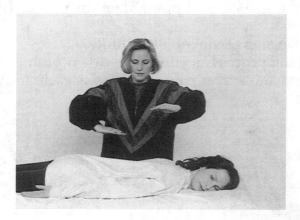

Fig. 6.2d

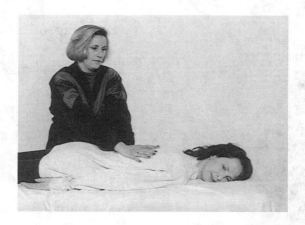

Fig. 6.2e

9) Have the person lie on his/her back once more. Apply a circular motion over the edge of the auric field, much the same as the rotation done previously. This rotation is done more gently, however, with the intent of "settling in" the energies. (Fig. 6.2f)
10) Now, gently touch each of the seven chakras from base to crown. (Fig. 6.2g)
11) Allow the client to get his/her bearings, and to sit up or stand when he/she feels fully ready. This is usually a very potent energy experience that takes a few moments for the recipient to assimilate.

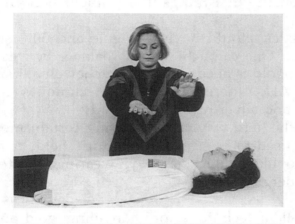

Fig. 6.2f

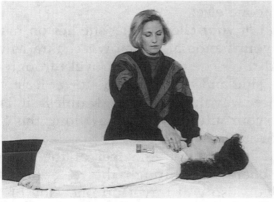

Fig. 6.2g

The Gold and Silver Rays

The *gold* ray is used for balancing masculine energy in a person, because gold embodies the masculine aspect of the Source. When infused in the body, this ray adds additional masculine energy that brings the recipient back into balance.

The *silver* ray is used for balancing feminine energy in a person, because silver embodies the feminine aspect of the Source. When infused in the body, this ray adds additional feminine energy that brings the recipient back into balance.

Males and females should have 50% gold and 50% silver in their auras. One can achieve this balance by wearing gold jewelry if gold is needed, and silver jewelry if silver is needed. Also, there are specific techniques for bringing the gold and silver rays into the body.

I have learned the hard way about wearing certain metals. Gold energy used to be scarce in my auric field. Unfortunately, I also liked silver jewelry; wearing it often unbalanced my energies.

This is an excellent technique for channeling gold and silver rays into someone else:

- Stand at the head of your client as he/she lies on his or her back. Place your hands at the crown chakra as you channel the gold ray. The color will travel through the body, down one side and up the other, for at least one revolution. Three revolutions is best, unless it isn't needed. Follow your intuition as to how long the gold energy should be applied.
- Next, place your hands upon the feet of the person. Send the silver energy up through the feet. Like the gold ray, the silver also will travel up one side of the

body and down the other as the gold does. Do the same amount of revolutions as the gold.

A variation of this technique is to have one person send gold energy through the crown, while another sends the silver ray through the feet. (Fig. 6.3) This is done simultaneously. As the gold is sent down the body, it is met by the silver traveling up the body. The two rays blend together as they balance the masculine/feminine energies in the person.

You can also apply this technique to yourself. In your meditations or as you are relaxing, visualize each ray as gold comes through your crown chakra while the silver ray travels up through your feet.

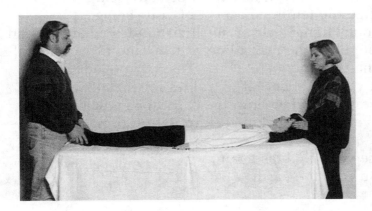

Fig. 6.3

The next exercise involves the innermost parts of you, your guides, and your Higher Self. Your Higher Self is the spiritual part of your essence. It links you with your other-dimensional selves and connects you with the Oversoul.* Your Higher Self is like a computer terminal; it links the rest of you to the mainframe or Oversoul.

---

* A large collection of Higher Selves

Merging the Gold and Silver Rays

- Balance the male and female energies by turning the chakras. (See Chapter 3 on Male/Female Balancing)
- Bring the gold ray through the crown chakra down to the heart chakra only. Move it at the heart in a clockwise direction.
- Bring the silver ray through the feet up to the heart chakra. Move it at the heart in a counter-clockwise direction.
- Feel your heart chakra open and expand.
- The two rays will begin to merge within your aura as they create a ley line grid* of energy.
- Visualize the masculine aspect of your being.
- Visualize the feminine aspect of your being.
- Ask your Higher Self or spiritual guides what gift can be brought to the masculine or feminine aspects to balance the two energies.
- Thank your Higher Self or guides for the answer.
- Release the ley lines into the earth for its healing.
- Bring your heart chakra back to its to normal open position.
- Balance your chakras again.
- Ground into the earth.

---

* See Chapter 14 for an in-depth explanation of the magnetic ley lines and the grids.

How to Relieve Trauma and Stress

Coping with stress and trauma seems to be part of everyday life in modern day western culture. Specific color rays relieve intense, stressful effects on your body, emotions, and mind. This exercise will fine tune your essence and bring it into a higher vibratory rate.

- Channel the *emerald* ray for healing. You may transmit it into one of the chakras or into the shoulders of the recipient. (Fig. 6.4a) It will go not only into his or her auric field, but also into the molecular and cellular structure of each of the bodies (physical as well as subtle).
- For those recipients needing to balance the masculine energy, input the *gold* ray into his or her shoulders. (also Fig. 6.4a) For those needing more feminine energy, channel the *silver* ray.
- Bring in the *lavender* ray for harmony, and transmit through the receiver's crown chakra. (Fig. 6.4b)

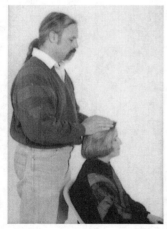
Fig. 6.4a

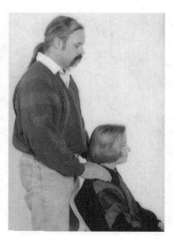
Fig. 6.4b

- As the healing channel, place your palms over the palms of the one receiving the healing. Send the *gold* ray and have the person transmute this energy by sending the *silver* ray back to you. (Fig. 6.4c) This will balance the masculine and feminine energies in his or her essence.

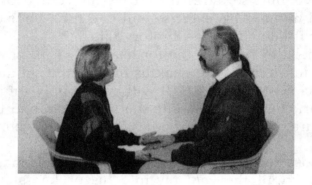

Fig 6.4.c

Chapter 7

Dealing with Psychic Hooks and Boundaries

"No one outside ourselves can rule us inwardly. When we know this, we become free."

---Buddha

Psychic hooks can be created without your conscious permission. They allow another to unconsciously steal your energy for the purpose of control. The need to do this may stem from a fear of loss.

A psychic hook, or cord, can definitely affect the physical body if left in place for any length of time. Initially, there is a drainoff of your energy resulting in fatigue. Eventually, the hook can adversely affect the chakra it is on or near, leading to disease in the nearby organs and systems of the body.

I have seen all kinds of psychic hooks. They have run the gamut from a less-lighted being who wished to control through what is termed "black magic", to one where the two involved truly loved each other but were very afraid of losing that love, resulting in a mutual psychic hook. I've also seen nearly everything in between.

A psychic hook typically looks like a dark brown or black cord, similar to a hose or rope. Of course, it can only be *seen* with psychic sight, but it can be felt in the auric field as a disturbance. It also can be perceived with *knowing* or clairaudience.

Generally, the color therapist allows the client to do his or her own recognizing, then cutting, of the psychic hook. Permitting a client to participate as much as possible in the process greatly empowers him or her; the therapist is merely a guide. If the client gets stuck, the therapist can facilitate the psychic hook removal process.

Psychic Hook Removal

An excellent technique for removing psychic hooks is:

- Have the person close his/her eyes and feel the body relax, like just before sleep.
- Have the person project his/her essence to that special place where the emotional body can be exclusively viewed.
- The person should "look" down upon his/her auric field. Discolorations in the emotional body will be apparent. These discolorations indicate potential psychic hooks.
- When a discoloration is discovered, "look" closely to see if there appears to be a hook in that area. Some discolorations do not contain hooks.
- If a hook is found, have the person trace it to its origin or owner. The hook is usually to another person (past or present). In some rare cases, it can even belong to another lifetime or dimension.
- To remove, the person should psychically cut the hook with an imaginary pair of gold scissors, then immediately take a small piece out of the hook to prevent it from reattaching easily. The small chunk should be wrapped in *pink* and *green* rays, then sent back to its owner with love and light, without hostility.

- Have the client tie off the cord where it leaves the body, as though it were an umbilical cord.
- Psychically take the pair of gold scissors and cut the cord near the tie.
- Send the dangling cord back to its owner with love and harmony, wrapped in the *rose* and *emerald* rays.
- See the tie and the hook, where it enters the body, shrivel up and drop off, just like a baby's an umbilical cord drops off after a couple of weeks.
- A void will be created where the psychic hook entered the body. Fill this void with rose and emerald rays. *This should be done several times over the next few days to insure that there is no reattachment.*
- When all psychic hooks have been cut, have the person bring his/her emotional self back into the body.

In some cases, the first couple of days following the psychic hook removal are shaky. Reattachment is still possible. The person should facilitate his or her personal empowerment through the use of the color rays. He/She should keep applying green and pink to the previously hooked spots to facilitate their detachment and healing. Since nature abhors a vacuum, filling the previously hooked spot with color is advisable. The processing of any emotions that may need to be expressed to prevent a reoccurrence is also necessary. Counseling or additional bodywork may be required to successfully do this. If the person is ambivalent about the cord, it may reconnect itself at any time, necessitating doing the technique again.

I find that psychic hooks vary from extremely negative energies to unintentionally harmful, but nevertheless needy, love connections. Most psychic hooks fall in the middle of those two zones. At any rate, they can be classified as a dysfunctional phenomenon, not mutually enhancing. Psychic hooks are dysfunctional because they are an integral part of a co-dependent relationship between the psychic hooker and the psychically hooked.

Monitoring Your Boundaries as a Healer or Psychic

You know that you are an empath. Your empathy is your blessing--and your curse. At least, it is your curse until you understand and put into practice the art of raising and lowering your boundaries at your command. You must be aware of what can harm your essence and watch your empathic powers like a hawk.

What is a boundary? It is a shield placed around your auric field which is composed of *white light* (protection), or the *13 rays* (for more heavy duty needs). It may be necessary to call on the *chrome ball* or the *lead shield* in unsafe areas. Simply visualize your auric field being shielded by a lead covering, similar to the lead shield the X-ray technician places on your body prior to taking X-rays. Another method is to picture yourself standing inside a large chrome ball of protection. Both of these protective devices can be lowered or raised at will, depending upon the environment in which you find yourself. It says "NO" to energies you do not wish to become a part of you. Of course, it may also be necessary to remove yourself physically from an unhealthy environment.

I frequently see "raving empaths" who have no conception of what, when, where, or how to begin to monitor the natural healing energies that spill from them.

Being an unconscious--or not consciously active--healer while refusing to admit your energy drainage can be unhealthy. Being an intense and active healer without doing the necessary energy monitoring can be lethal.

71

Realize that you are a healer *at all times*, even during your sleep or so-called rest periods. I have, as have others, spent many nights engaged in personal, planetary, and interdimensional "running" of the color rays.

During these times, I have been energetically jerked out of my body by Gaia (the spiritual goddess consciousness of the planet Earth) and sent into fault lines ready to erupt into an earthquake. I've helped souls transition from Earth to the next realm of existence. I have spent significant amounts of time healing and teaching on other levels of existence. You, too, have probably performed these tasks for Spirit.

Even though our Higher Selves may agree to this, the impact on the physical body is not always taken into account. I call this the "Mack Truck Syndrome"--feeling as though you have been run over by a Mack truck when you awaken in the morning! There needs to be a careful consideration of the body's needs in this work...<u>All</u> of the bodies: physical, emotional, mental, and spiritual. The Higher Self usually understands the toll that the earth experience takes on a person; it will use divine discernment as to when healing is appropriate and when it is not. Sometimes, the Higher Self will make a risky decision for the greater good, even if it temporarily impacts the physical body.

If you are emotionally or mentally unstable or out of balance, or if your physical body is sick--<u>don't</u> do any healing or psychic work. Your conscious, physical personality is empowered to tell your Higher Self, "Enough already! I am off duty tonight. I need some relaxation time to recoup my energy. I will let you know when I am ready to do more healing work."

Other people will recognize that you have the special capability of bringing forth the energy of Creation, something that they may desperately need more of. Some people are simply needy, others are "energy vampires". The boundaries you create will monitor your energy system and keep it from being drained. You are no good to anyone if you are burned out. You cannot heal or help everyone on this planet; many do not even want healing. No <u>one</u> person can do it all. Better to have many good years as a productive, happy, and healthy healer than to have a short, out-of-control lifetime where the world loses a good lightworker through burnout or death.

Monitor your electromagnetic field, particularly after being with others. Often, you may feel depressed, or angry, or sad when the feelings aren't even your own; you may have unconsciously picked up the energy of another person and incorporated it into your own aura. To leave yourself fully open by not monitoring your boundaries is to give yourself away to <u>any</u> and <u>all</u>. This creates gaping holes in your auric field; holes which make you vulnerable to psychic hooks and energy possession by others.

Realize that your boundaries are disrupted when you are attached to the outcome of your help. Don't set up a karmic situation of codependency and possible psychic hooks. Don't go into the healing with specific expectations for the person desiring the healing; rather approach them with unconditional love and with a professionally detached manner.

Your boundaries are also disturbed when you have alcohol and drug dependencies. These addictions punch holes in your auric field. When you don't care about yourself (due to lack of balance or low self-esteem), you have no idea what your limits or boundaries are. You can no longer psychically defend yourself.

Realize that the ability to perfectly monitor your boundaries as a healer isn't mastered overnight. It is an ongoing process of checks and balances. Perhaps, that is why most of us don't immediately have access to the full range of our abilities; it is something we develop and work with as we go along. If we did have all of our powers immediately, would we then have the wisdom to use them with discernment? I believe that our abilities unfold <u>after</u> we gain better balance and wisdom.

Obtaining Permission for Healing

In Chapter 5, I briefly touched on the necessity for getting permission to do any healing work on another person. The importance of this should not be underestimated. Healing energy can always be sent to the soul or Higher Self. However, conscious permission needs to be obtained if healing energy is sent to the physical, emotional, or mental bodies.

If permission is not granted, the healer may become part of the karmic cycle belonging to the person who is ill. This is the way it works: For whatever reason, the ill person has manifested the condition. Of course, he or she can change this. Sometimes the individual feels that he or she is discharging a karmic debt. Karma is the universal law of balance, or cause and effect. In other words, for every action there is a reaction. Often, the illness or disease is manifested as a result of low self-esteem or selfworth. The person feels he/she deserves to be ill. By sending non-requested healing energy, you have meddled in whatever soul-imposed lesson is taking place. Then it involves you. Why take on unnecessary karma by violating the universal law of free will?

There are two basic ways one may get permission for a healing:
1. Ask the person consciously, "May I send you healing energy (for that physical, emotional, or mental condition)?" Healing for any body, except the spiritual, requires specific permission from the individual.

2. Ask the Higher Self of the person, "Does this person really want healing energy (for his/her physical, emotional or mental condition)?" You may always send healing energy specifically to the soul or Higher Self, then it can distribute the energy as it sees fit. If you are specifically asking permission of the Higher Self to heal the other bodies, be sure you are in tune with that particular Higher Self, and that you are getting accurate information.

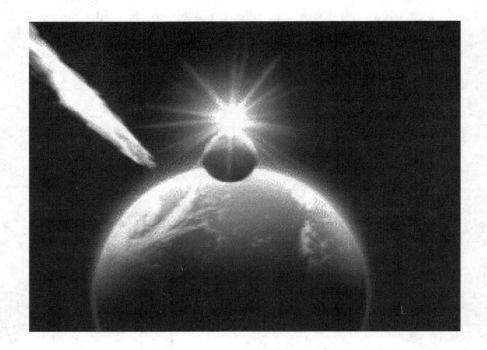

Chapter 8
Chakra Blocks

═══════════════════════════

You

You are the Light

You are the Dawn

You are the Doorway

You are the One

---Omega
July 1991

When you open the heart chakra, you are opening to the divinity within you and your connection to the divinity in others. You begin to recognize that through the Love energy of Creation we are all linked to one another.

If your heart chakra is partially or completely shut down, you've probably been emotionally traumatized or wounded; you've tried to protect yourself from what you perceive as more disappointment or hurt. Often this common reaction works in the reverse by trapping the fear and pain in the chakra. This can occur in childhood or adulthood. One can even bring blockages into the body from other lifetimes.

Opening your heart chakra will not open you to more pain or disillusionment, but will actually allow the healing process to occur, freeing you to experience deeper levels of Love. You may initially feel vulnerable, but understanding precedes healing, making it easier to allow the heart chakra to open.

A practical reason for opening the heart chakra is to use it to transmit healing energy. The heart is a very powerful way to send healing energy to others, sometimes more effective than the hands-on approach.

Opening the Heart Chakra

- Work with a partner.
- Greet one another: "From the God of my being to the God of your being, in Light, Love, harmony, and balance." Your hands are in the *pronam* (prayer-like) position. (Fig. 8.1a)
- Place your hand upon the heart chakra of the other. You will send either the *emerald* ray or the *rose* ray into the heart of the other person. Color will come

through your hand to form a special bond with your partner. (Fig. 8.1b)

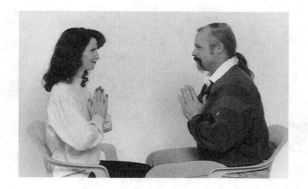

Fig 8.1a

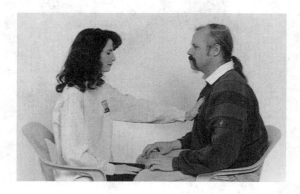

Fig. 8.1b

- Place one of your palms against the palm of your partner, touching (with the fingers) first the forehead of
  one, then the other. (Fig. 8.1c and Fig. 8.1d)

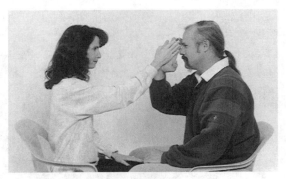

Fig. 8.1c

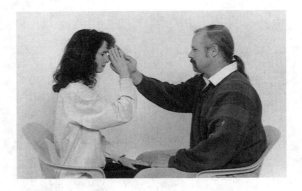

Fig. 8.1d

Chakra Blockages

The heart chakra is not the only energy center in the body that can be closed down or resistant to its full expression. All of the chakras are subject to our issues and our traumas. I have reason to believe these blockages often germinate from the seeds of past lives or current life experiences. Especially hard hit is the throat chakra, the communication center of the body, along with the solar plexus chakra, the center of power, ego, and self-love. For many people, there has been much societal and familial resistance to speaking their truth. This is linked to feelings of low self-esteem, and frequently to abuse of their power energy.

The color healer can do much to facilitate the clearing of the blocked areas within the chakra system. When such a chakra is being worked on, you should always try to discover the cause of the block, and how best to eliminate it. This may entail some spiritual counseling or dialogue between you and the other person to uncover the deeper reasons for the block. An effective method for ascertaining the problem area is the Causal Plane technique described in Chapter 14.

Always attempt to get to the *root cause* of an energetic imbalance or block. Not uncovering the mental, emotional, or spiritual misalignment will generally render the healing ineffective.

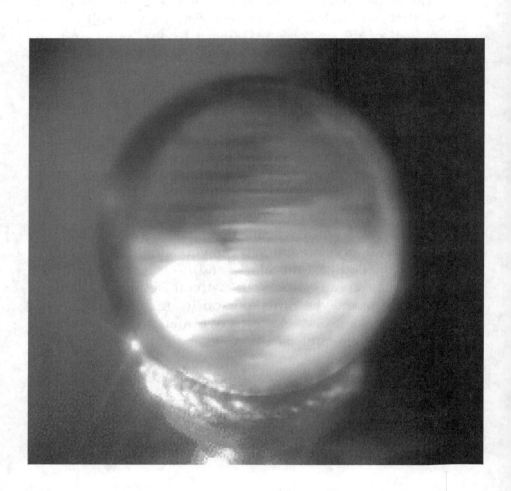

Chapter 9

Crystals, Herbs, and Color

==

Crystals of Movement

Flowers of Light

Crystals of Movement

Sounds that are bright

Colors in attunement

---Korton
August 1991

Other effective forms of balancing the chakras include the use of crystals and herbs.

The emphasis of a crystal should be on its color, as well as its potential usefulness for a certain problem. It's the opposite with herbs; we are looking primarily for the healing properties of each plant, not just the particular color as many herbal colors are similar earth shades. Sometimes, however, color is a key factor in choosing both herbs and crystals.

The crystal kingdom is both physical and etheric. In contrast, herbs are very physical and earth-oriented in their nature. Both elements balance the chakras very well; it is up to you which you feel drawn to use.

There are many crystals and gemstones that are often appropriate. I will name just a few. If you wish to delve more deeply into crystal healing, you should read some of the many books on crystals. I recommend the series of books by Katrina Raphaell: <u>Crystal Enlightenment</u>, <u>Crystal Healing</u>, and <u>The Crystalline Transmission</u>. Another wonderful book is Melody's <u>Love is in the Earth: A Kaleidoscope of Crystals</u>.

There are many viewpoints on how to clean crystals. I council practitioners to use their intuition regarding crystal clearing. Some crystal experts say no physical cleaning is necessary; simply allow crystals to air for a few hours.

For those who choose to clean their crystals following their application, place them on a plate with sea salt or Epsom salts. Another method for cleaning is to soak them in a mixture of 1/3 part apple cider vinegar, 1/3 part sea salt, and 2/3 part warm water. You may also use the ocean to clean your crystals.

Caution: Some crystals cannot withstand water or other solutions without crumbling or discoloring. Other crystals are adversely affected by salts. Check with your rock shop or gem store for help on this.

Crystals

First chakra	Ruby, garnet, bloodstone, red jasper
Second chakra	Orange topaz, amber, carnelian, orange adventurine, orange calcite
Third chakra	Wulfenite, citrine, yellow topaz, apatite, sulfur, yellow fluorite
Fourth chakra (Green aspect)	Dioptase, green tourmaline, emerald, peridot, green adventurine, jade
Fourth chakra (Rose aspect)	Pink tourmaline, kunzite, rose quartz, lapidolyte
Fifth chakra	Aquamarine, blue topaz, celestite, crysocolla, turquoise, angelite
Sixth chakra	Lapis, sodalite, azurite
Seventh chakra	Amethyst, sugilite, purple fluorite, lavender quartz
Eighth chakra	Silver, galena, hematite
Ninth chakra	Gold, pyrite, yellow amber
Tenth chakra	White quartz, pearl, white opal, selenite
Eleventh chakra	Diamond, clear quartz, natural silicon
Twelfth chakra	Black obsidian, onyx, black pearl

Balancing the Chakras With Crystals

One of my favorite methods for balancing the chakras is:
• Have the person lie down on his or her back.
• Place your sensing hand over the base chakra. Focus on the energy of the base chakra. As you begin to perceive the flow, you can tell if there is an imbalance or a difficulty in this region.
• Place one of the base chakra stones in your transmitting hand while you hold your sensing hand over the chakra. Perceive the energy flow in the chakra as you

hold each stone, one at a time. With the appropriate stone, you will feel an intensity in the energy flow.

- Once you determine which stone is appropriate for the base chakra, you will then place the stone on the chakra for balancing. Stay attuned to the auric field until you feel the energy pattern has shifted to normal. It should take only a few minutes.
- Do this with each of the other chakras, ending with the crown.

Herbs

First chakra	Ginseng, damiana, garlic
Second chakra	Black cohosh, pennyroyal, nettle
Third chakra	Yarrow, blessed thistle, cinnamon
Fourth chakra (Green aspect)	Juniper berries, sandalwood, pinion pine
Fourth chakra (Rose aspect)	Rosehips, cumin, lavender
Fifth chakra	Bladderack (kelp), cayenne, mullein
Sixth chakra	Eyebright, fennel, feverfue
Seventh chakra	Jasmine, sarsaparilla, gotu kola
Eighth chakra	Valerian, passion flower, bloodroot
Ninth chakra	Coltsfoot, goldenseal, cleavers
Tenth chakra	White willow bark, sage, white mushroom
Eleventh chakra	Bayberry, cedar, astrogalus
Twelfth chakra	Black walnut, barberry, devil's claw

Balancing the Chakras With Herbs

Use a small amount of the herb (a couple of ounces) placed in a small bag, preferably made of a natural cloth fiber.

- Have the person lie down on his or her back.

- Place one hand over the base chakra. Focus on the energy of the base chakra. As you begin to perceive the flow, you can tell if there is an imbalance or a difficulty in this region.
- Place one of the base chakra herbs in your transmitting hand, while you hold your sensing hand over the chakra. Perceive the energy flow in the chakra as you hold each herb, one at a time. With the appropriate herb, you will feel an intensity in the energy flow.
- Once you determine which herb is appropriate for the base chakra, place the herb on the chakra for balancing. Stay attuned to the auric field until you feel the energy pattern has shifted to normal. It will take only a few minutes.
- Do this with each of the other chakras, ending with the crown.

Other Methods of Healing With Color

Besides the hands-on methods, there are many ways to work with color healing. A high-voltage lamp covered with a specific color filter provides a slower, but effective, means of transmitting color energy. Hand-held devices like the LED light which emits a soothing--yet potent--light beam, can be most beneficial.

Shades of colors that are compatible with your auric field can enhance or heal your electromagnetic field. This is also a form of color healing. The wearing of certain colors, or decorating your surroundings in your personal color hues is a variation of this idea. (See Chapter 1)

Other methods involve the use of water, the Sun, or the Moon as they provide particular frequencies of light.

Magnetizing Water

Water is also a carrier of the unconscious. Just as the Moon (which according to the ancient Earth religions is a reflection of our feminine energy and our subconscious) affects the ocean tides, so it affects us as well, for we, like the great seas, are composed primarily of water.

• Hold a glass of water in your sensing hand.
• Channel energy (emerald green is a good color) through your transmitting hand, into the water.
• The water is now charged with healing energy, so drink up!

Solarizing Water

You can also "lunarize" water by doing the same process using the light of a full Moon.

• Place a glass or pan of water in the sunlight.
• Put a color swatch upon the glass. The Sun will radiate that color into the water. Leave it out for a least a day.
• By drinking the water, you will be consuming that color vibration.

Clearing Tap Water

In my opinion, the quality of most tap water is questionable. The water boards claim that our drinking water is "perfectly safe", even with chlorine added.* I have a strong sensitivity to tap water, and learned early on to eliminate it from my diet.

- Place your sending hand over the glass.
- Channel red, orange, yellow, and black until it "feels" complete.
- Your water is now drinkable. It may still taste as if it has chlorine in it, but I have found that, within my own body, the harmful effects are neutralized. I do not get a "chlorine reaction" consisting of a constant headache and malaise. (You can improve the taste of tap water by running the green ray.)

---

* In spite of the "official line", the 1992 <u>American Journal of Public Health</u> reported the combined results of 10 studies linking chlorinated drinking water with increases in the rates of rectal and bladder cancer. The findings came from researchers at Harvard University and the Medical College of Wisconsin.

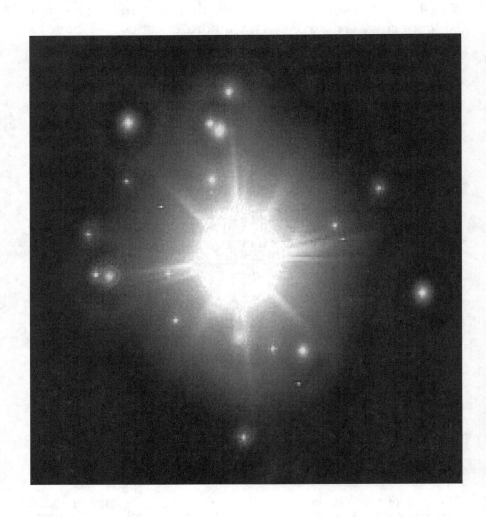

Chapter 10

The Clearing Process

The Search

A solitary physical being
Confused and terribly alone

Reaching for a source
That exists in some unknown

Finding a link, a color
A sound
Touching tomorrow, union is found

---Thor
July 1991

Planetary Clearings

What if you were suddenly plucked off Earth and sub-sequently deposited upon a planet that vibrated at a higher rate, such as a 4th dimensional vibration? What do you think would happen to each of your bodies--physical, emotional, mental, and spiritual?

Imagine continuous shocks of energy 100,000 times stronger than those you are used to!

What if there was misalignment in your physical, emotional, and mental bodies? What would happen to your physical body's problems? They would all be triggered at once!

If your emotional body had what my teachers call the "four deadly sins" (greed, ego, fear, and adultery) or other misalignments, they also would be triggered.

Any mental blockages would apply unbearable pressure to your mental processes affected by the energy. How would you handle the numerous negative thoughts that would come up all at once? How would your limited thinking be "stretched" to accept a very different, tele-pathic, and symbiotic lifestyle?

The final result would be illness or death of the physi-cal body, severe emotional instability, mental confusion, or insanity. Unless, of course, you have cleared all of your bodies and aligned your "past" or simultaneous lifetimes.

What does all this mean?

To *live* on the 4th dimension, we must be *ready* for the 4th dimension. Any areas that have not been cleared or aligned will prevent us from existing in this elevated vi-bration comfortably.

We are told by our guides that Source has decided to elevate all of Creation approximately one dimension and a half. As I write this, we on Earth currently exist in the middle of the 3rd dimension. That means that the 3rd dimension will eventually be elevated into the 4th dimension or higher. Each subsequent dimension will also graduate a dimension and a half, not only on Earth, but across all of Creation. My spirit guides have told me that Creation will never again be this vibrationally dense.

The 3rd dimension is a point of tension, providing the movement that this change will take. We call this the "rubberband effect". This is the only dimension where the dualities (good and evil) exist side-by-side; hence, the friction.

On the 4th dimension there is telepathy...spiritually-attuned people and spiritually-unattuned people remain at opposite ends of the universe; it is very uncomfortable for them to mingle. Because they keep themselves separate, it is difficult to increase the level of tension within their civilizations.

In the lighter dimensions there is symbiosis, resulting in a harmonious, tension-free existence.

Thus, this manifest world has shown itself to be an important key. It provides enough tension to create movement, for itself as well as the other dimensions. For many incarnations we physically clothed spirit beings felt we were participating in a dress rehearsal on the stage of life. We now know that the practice is finished and we are creatively "playing the play"--the intent of which is to truly bridge Spirit and matter.

As we become more aligned, we distance ourselves from the opposite, darker polarity, that which misuses energy and is into controlling everything. This creates the rubberband effect. In the process, tension stretches the two polarities until they snap. The snap will propel us into a vibration that is less dense.

The clearing processes contribute to the tension. They are stimulated by waves of energy from the Source, or

God. These waves will continue to be cyclic until the new level of vibration is in effect.

In a sense, this process of tension and release could be likened to the birth of a baby, or a sexual climax. Both are processes that will happen regardless; there is no going back once it's begun. This is also true regarding the massive amount of energy coming from the Source.

To make the transition into the 4th dimension, my guides have told me that we must have approximately 25% of the planet's population "aware and caring" about the Earth. Their actions towards their earthbound brothers and sisters should reflect such spiritual growth. This will be sufficient to affect the changes necessary for the people of Earth, so they can begin to live together in harmony, understanding, and peace.

The Harmonic Convergence in August 1987 signaled the start of the much needed clearing processes and releasing of blocks. This first wave was the **physical** clearing of our physical bodies. The intensity of the wave peaked in March of 1988. During that time there were certain diseases that became more widespread. These included candida, the Epstein-Barr virus, Chronic Fatigue Syndrome, and AIDS. All of these are directly associated with a compromise of the body's immune system. That which needs to be cleared within the chakras is directly connected to the immune/endocrine system. When one succumbs to one of these problems, the immune system has been weakened, often from the clearing process.

I've been asked whether one *has* to get sick to clear. Hopefully, not. Imbalances seem to occur in your weakest link, the body with which you are the least comfortable.

If you are less identified with your physical body, it may be the one that gets out of balance the easiest. Also, if you don't properly care for the physical body, it is more likely to feel the stress from the clearings.

Body	Initial Entry	Exit	Next Entry	Exit
Physical	August 1987	March 1988	August 1994	March 1995
Cellular	August 1988	March 1989	August 1995	March 1996
Emotional	August 1989	March 1990	August 1996	March 1997
Mental	August 1990	March 1991	August 1997	March 1998
Spiritual	August 1991	March 1994	August 1998	March 2001

Chart 10-1

The next wave of energy to impact the physical body came in August of 1994, peaking in March of 1995. At this time, the energy was amplified by 100,000 times (in comparison to the first time it came in 1987).

The second wave came in August 1988 (the anniversary of the Harmonic Convergence) and lasted until March 1989. It affected **cellular** clearing (the release of blocks in the cellular body), the DNA/RNA coding that comes from our ancestors. When you totally clear this body, you also clear it for your family. Unbelievable? Yes, but it works. If you should get a disease following total clearing and processing of the cellular body, it won't be due to your family pattern. It will result from something you have done to yourself, or from toxins found in your environment.

The next wave of energy to impact the cellular body will arrive in August of 1995; it will peak in March of 1996. At this time, the energy will amplify by 100,000 times (compared to the first time it came in 1988).

The third wave heralding the **emotional** clearing arrived in August 1989 and lasted until March 1990. Extreme moods, along with throat and chest problems, were rampant during this process. Males, in general, have more challenges during waves of emotional clearing than females. Most males on this planet are less comfortable with their emotions; thus, they have a more difficult time acknowledging that they even <u>have</u> an emotional body!

The next wave of energy to impact the emotional body will arrive in August of 1996; it will peak in March of 1997. At this time, the energy will amplify by 100,000 times (compared to the first time it came in 1989).

The **mental** body clearing began in August 1990 and lasted until March 1991. Mental confusion, dyslexia (even for people who'd never before had it), frequent headaches, and TMJ (muscle/joint tightness in the jaw) were common ailments associated with this cleansing. Females, in general, had more problems with this clearing than males. Unless the female was particularly mental, she probably had more challenges than did her male counterparts.

The next wave of energy to impact the mental body will arrive in August of 1997; it will peak in March of 1998. At this time, the energy will amplify by 100,000 times (compared to the first time it came in 1990).

The wave of **simultaneous lifetimes alignment** started in August 1991 and ran until March of 1994. This process entailed alignment with all your "past" lives, or what I usually refer to as simultaneous lives. Truly, there is no such thing as past or future, only the present, or the eternal NOW.

For convenience, we have agreed, at this physical reality, to a linear systematic framing of space and time. All that we are, including our simultaneous lifetimes, is there to be assimilated. All of our knowledge and experience is incorporated into our "present" existence to draw on as we need it. We experience our simultaneous lifetimes alignment process through vivid dreams, and déjà vu feelings. In a similar way to the other clearings, we process our simultaneous lifetimes through our physical, emotional, and mental bodies.

Duality energy has always been magnified the most at the densest physical level (the 3rd dimension). In April

96

1991, a New Age spiritual-oriented group I attended held an active meditation/exercise to bring the yin and yang energy together. That meditation, along with the subsequent "11:11"* event, the solar and lunar eclipse, and the alignment of planets in 1991, helped tremendously in the amplification of the energy. After this occurrence, we noticed a distinct upsurge in the clearing energies.

This new tension has had a two-edged effect: on the one hand, it is speeding-up the positive effects upon humanity and the Earth; on the other, it is applying incredible pressure upon all weak or unaligned areas. It is literally forcing clearing. *"Lightworkers"* (people dedicated to spreading the Light and Love of Source) are probably feeling it the most, as their energy systems remain open to changes from the Source. The positive effects include new ways of working through our perceived differences...to discover our commonalties, to find ways to treat each other with respect, to show love and concern for the earth, and to align our souls within our bodies, without blocks.

The next wave of energy to impact the simultaneous lifetimes alignment will arrive in August of 1998; it will peak in March of 2001. At this time, the energy will amplify by 100,000 times (compared to the first time it came in 1991).

On July 26, 1992, in the midst of the active simultaneous lifetimes alignment process, Creation opened yet another doorway. The intense light of the Source "beamed down" the red ray. For a six-week period, the red ray colored our clearing processes, bringing strong physical en-

---

* The date January 11, 1992 in numerology is a vibration of "11:11". Its significance is that it is a doorway through which there is an activation of the energy from Creation. There will be on-going, activated "gates" from time to time.

ergy with an emphasis on grounding, survival, bones and muscles, and base chakra issues.

Each six week period then saw an infusion of the next rainbow ray in the color sequence. As the previous ray faded out, another was focused on Earth.

The doorways are openings for incoming energies, stepped-up for the needed Earth clearings. This chart shows the rays of color that will be emphasized during these six-week periods. (See Chart 10-2) You may draw on their particular energies for clearing yourself.

The Doorways of Energy Intensity

Color	Initial Entry Date	Next Entry Date
Red	July 26, 1992	July 26, 1999
Orange	September 6, 1992	September 6, 1999
Yellow	October 18, 1992	October 18, 1999
Green	November 29, 1992	November 29, 1999
Rose	January 10, 1993	January 10, 2000
Translucent Blue	February 21, 1993	February 21, 2000
Indigo	April 4, 1993	April 4, 2000
Violet	May 16, 1993	May 16, 2000
Silver	June 27, 1993	June 27, 2000
Gold	August 8, 1993	August 8, 2000
White	September 19, 1993	September 19, 2000
Clear	October 31, 1993	October 31, 2000
Black	December 12, 1993	December 12, 2000

Chart 10-2

Each color ray has its own emphasis or consciousness, issues, and traits that will be projected during its particular time period, giving us the opportunity to clear and incorporate it within us. (See Chart 2-1 to clarify the impact each ray has on particular parts of the body.)

With the completion of the black ray in January 1994, the date of February 2, 1994 confirmed the entry of the "rainbow energy". The collective energy did not escalate between that time and the beginning of the physical clearing cycle in August 1994. It was, however, a time of rest, a time to process the shifts and adjustments needed after multiple clearings. The rainbow energy suffuses all of your bodies, all aspects of your life are highlighted for the clearing process.

On December 12, 1994, the "12:12" gateway was opened. Its planetary effect was to amplify the male/female energies within each person, and impact more strongly those who have not cleared as deeply.

Ways to Facilitate Physical Clearing

- Epsom salt baths
- Bodywork such as massage, chiropractic, acupuncture
- Drinking sufficient pure water
- Proper healthful diet
- Sufficient exercise
- Sufficient rest and relaxation
- Minimizing stress-producing aspects
- Avoiding toxic environments

Cellular Cleansing Technique

- Work with a partner. Sit facing each other.
- Place a protective beam of white light around both of you.
- Together, bring forth the *green* energy from the earth into your right hands and hold it.
- Both partners bring forth the *rose* ray of love from Creation. Hold the ray in your left hands.
- Designate who will send the energy first. As the sender, move both of your hands over your partner's auric field. As you move over the electromagnetic field, your hands will signal shifts in energy. These are points on your partner's body that would benefit from direct touch as you project the rays into these areas. Repeat until all is clear and flowing. You may also receive pictures or thoughts regarding specific lives or experiences of the other person. Please share these with him/her.
- Now, have your partner be the sender. Repeat the process.
- Release the rays. Ground yourselves with the *silver* and *gold* rays. Clear!

Facilitating Emotional Clearing

Feelings reflected most often in the emotional clearing:
- Anger
- Fear
- Intense sorrow

Ways the emotions express:
- Body Illness

- Personality (out of the ordinary behavior or traits)
- Intense expression of the emotions themselves

Emotional Clearing Using Crystals and Gemstones

Condition	Crystal or Gemstone	Direction Along Body
Emotions clearing through the physical body (toxins, heavy metals)	Ruby	*Down* the spine or whole body
Emotions clearing in the first stage (which mostly affects the physical body)	Emerald or green tourma-line	*Down* the spine or whole body
Emotions clearing in the second stage emotional/spiritual level, that which doesn't express through your physical body. Intangible.	Rose quartz or kunzite	*Up* the spine

Facilitating Mental Clearing

Exercise 1: Blending Rays

Purpose: Clears mental debris, facilitates healing, brain synaptical clearing, brain synaptical connecting (within the "tensor" or psychic centers in the brain)
- Bring the *emerald green, translucent blue, indigo,* and *violet* rays simultaneously through your crown chakra. (This combination will form a wine color.)
- As you bring them in, focus on the tensor centers of the brain, located about 4/5's of the way inside your brain's interior (no function of that area is scientifically known at this time).
- Allow the blended colors to expand.

- Keep expanding until your head becomes tight.
- At this point, allow the blended rays to flow down to the heart center, then release them out into the earth.

Exercise 2: The Pen Technique

Purpose: Healing dyslexic symptoms produced by mental clearing. Facilitates balance between both halves of the brain.
- Place your feet firmly on the floor, grounding to the earth.
- Bring the *gold* ray into your crown chakra and the *silver* ray up through your feet simultaneously. This will balance your male/female energies.
- Take a pen in hand (held vertically) and place about a foot in front of you. (A pen or pencil is light, narrow, and convenient to use.)
- Keeping your eyes on the pen, slowly move it in a circular path to one side until you can no longer see it.
- Move it back towards the center, then to the other side (in the same manner) until you can no longer see it.
- Repeat two more times.
- Return to the center position, switching the pen to a horizontal position in your hand. Follow the pen with your eyes as you lift it upwards, until you can no longer see it. Then move it downwards until it cannot be seen.
- Repeat two more times.

Exercise 3: The Blank Screen Technique

Purpose: This technique helps you connect with your mental processes, past and present.

- Ground to the earth. Your feet should be flat on the floor, and your eyes should be closed.
- In a relaxed manner, focus on your 3rd eye. See a blank screen behind your closed eyelids.
- Allow the mind to be still. Just be the observer.
- As you passively look at the screen, you may see miscellaneous pictures. Do not attempt to control, just quietly observe.
- Remain in this mode for 5 minutes. Do this daily for a period of one week. You may increase to 10 minutes a day the second week, then 15 minutes a day during the third week.

Questions To Ask Yourself

- What lives are attached to my mental clearing?
- Is there something that I am presently doing that belongs to another mental experience?

Simultaneous Lifetimes Alignment

The simultaneous lifetimes process is your assimilation of "past life" data. This data assimilates directly into your physical body, primarily at the head, in the pineal and pituitary glands.

This technique will facilitate you as the data from your simultaneous lifetimes is assimilated. It will increase the capacity of the pineal and pituitary glands to process the information psychically.

- Locate the pituitary gland in the center of the brain, across from the third eye. It is connected to the 6th chakra.

- Locate the pineal gland. (It is a few inches behind the pituitary gland, and a little higher.) The pineal gland is connected to the crown, or 7th chakra.
- Bring forth the *violet* ray from the Source, into your crown chakra, and send it to your pineal gland. Fill it with the violet energy. The pineal gland is also violet, so it is similar to placing "violet upon violet" until it is a deep purple.
- Beam the violet ray from the pineal gland to the pituitary gland. Fill the pituitary with violet energy. It will appear as indigo changing into violet.
- Next, run the violet ray from the pituitary out the 3rd eye back to Source. You have effectively created a triangle.
- Keep the violet ray running in this triangle formation for at least 2 or 3 minutes. Your head may feel as if it's expanding; there may even be some vibration.
- Now, release the energy.
- Re-ground yourself.

Clearing and Assimilating Simultaneous Lives

Purpose: To clear and assimilate the events, lessons, and data of your "past" lives.

- In your imagination, create a rainbow consisting of all 13 color rays.
- Bring this rainbow in through your crown chakra, flowing down to the base chakra. Circle the base chakra 13 times to the left, then 13 times to the right.
- Move the rainbow up to the spleen chakra. Circle it there 13 times in each direction.
- Do this at the solar plexus, heart, throat, third eye, and crown.
- Send the rainbow out of your crown chakra like a fountain of light, directed at both palm chakras simultaneously. Move the rainbow 13 times to the left around the palm chakras, then 13 times to the right.
- Focus the rainbow out of the palms into the earth below your feet (about 6 inches). Move it 13 times to the left, 13 to the right.
- Bring the rainbow up from the earth, through your feet, along the spinal column, past the crown (about 6 inches above the head). Again, rotate it 13 times in each direction.
- Spray the rainbow colors (like a fountain) down the auric field, past the feet again, then back up the body. Repeat this a total of 13 times.
- This exercise encompasses all of the chakras, both physical and non-physical.
- Re-ground.

Life Force Energy

When we are born, we have 100% of our life force energy. This can be depleted immediately, or over time. Oriental medicine teaches that you cannot regain life force energy; you have to rely on what is called *defensive energy*. This rule is no longer true.

Defensive energy corresponds to the immune system. It helps to maintain our internal environment as it battles against external forces that would harm it.

In the past, with Earth's denser vibrations, you couldn't clear and align all four of your bodies; reaching Source consciousness was nearly impossible. It was too difficult to get past the denseness, to finally touch spiritual consciousness.

For the first time since the fall of Atlantis and Lemuria (two ancient civilizations on the earth), eons ago, you have the opportunity to regain your lost life-force energy. However, without preparation, the average person cannot do so. There are several key elements involved in this process. All four of your bodies must be clear and aligned; you have to work not only with the energy of Creation but with the energy of Earth, connecting to them in a balanced, androgynous way. *In this state, you operate in the world, with unlimited, balanced energy, even halting the aging process.* As long as you are in a state of duality, you cannot regain your lost life-force energy.

Begin with the basics I gave you earlier in this book. Practice them faithfully on a daily basis. Practical application of the other exercises in this book will facilitate necessary clearing and aligning processes. They will help you reach the state of Source and Earth connectedness required for these special states of being.

Chapter 11

The Responsibilities of a Healer

"Now we see through a glass, darkly; but then face to face: now I know in part; but then shall know even as also I am known."

---The Bible
1 Corinthians 13-12

Self-Evaluation

This is a self-evaluation of your state of being at this time. Please list a minimum of four things that you do for yourself in each area:

Physical

Diet

1. _____

2. _____

3. _____

4. _____

Exercise

1. _____

2. _____

3. _____

4. _____

Playtime

1. _____

2. _____

3. _____

4. _____

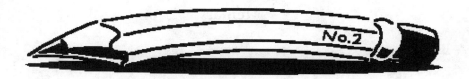

Emotional

<u>Meditation</u>

1. _____

2. _____

3. _____

4. _____

<u>Counseling</u>

1. _____

2. _____

3. _____

4. _____

<u>Support Groups</u>

1. _____

2. _____

3. _____

4. _____

Mental

<u>Reading</u>

1. _____

2. _____

3. _____

4. _____

<u>Mentally-oriented games</u>

1. _____

2. _____

3. _____

4. _____

<u>Work</u>

1. _____

2. _____

3. _____

4. _____

Spiritual

1. _____

2. _____

3. _____

4. _____

How does one "grade" the little test or evaluation you have just completed? There are no grades; there are only weak or strong areas. These will show you where more work is needed to achieve balance and alignment.

You may ask, why is this self-evaluation called "Responsibilities of a Healer?"

Webster defines <u>responsibility</u> as "being accountable for one's behavior or action." I would like to offer another definition. To me, responsibility means the "ability to respond," the willingness to **respond** to others in a balanced, aligned way, rather than simply **reacting**. So, how does this pertain to us?

Reaction, in my definition, implies an unconscious triggering stimulus, one that is not thought out. For example: We often see people who seem to be in a "closed loop" regarding their interactions with others. They are "triggered" to react in an angry, defensive, or victimized way to something someone says or does. Their current behavior has more to do with past patterns (set up in childhood), from earlier dysfunctional relationships.

Response, on the other hand, implies integrity to self, that one is responsible to all four of his/her bodies. Even Webster defines response as being likened to responsibility, answerable to something whether it be positive or negative.

The process of self-realization involves response and responsibility. Self-realization means that your thoughts, feelings, actions, and perceptions are **internally** generated, although they may be triggered by external stimuli. It means having an equal regard for all of your bodies. It means seeing the importance of physical health, mental flexibility, emotional fluidity, spiritual acceptance, and harmony between all your bodies. A self-realized person has no expectations or judgments regarding his/her inter-actions with others; one is involved with the process, not the outcome. Remember, at any given time, we have a choice in how we respond.

In the process of facilitating healing, responsibility is very important. **The responsibilities of a healer involve:**

• Knowing that a healer is only a facilitator.
• Being as aligned as possible at that point in his/her evolution.
• Knowing when another healer/practitioner will do a better job of facilitating a particular person, then refer-ring the person to him or her.
• Being willing to put your own issues aside, so that you may facilitate healing for someone else.
• Being willing to clear your issues.

Now, I wish to state something which may seem irrev-erent to some. **GOD DOES NOT HEAL YOU, YOU HEAL YOURSELF.**[*]

You are solely responsible for the choices you have made in your life and in your health. You are a part of

---

[*] I am, however, a firm believer in the power of prayer as a healing source. Dr. Larry Dossey has shown in his research into the myriad studies of prayer, that it is an incredible tool for transformation. It can rise above belief systems of all kinds, affect amoeba in petrie dishes, and even transcend the time continuum! Prayer seems to be a force that is not circumscribed by any religion or boxed in to any par-ticular emotional or mental belief constructs.

God, and because of this you were given free will to make your own decisions. Will you respond to the Divinity within you, or choose more or less to ignore it?

Long Distance Healing

Color energy is great for short or long distance healing. Light and Love know no boundaries, a convenient fact when you are physically not present with the person you want to work on.

Long distance healing is not dissimilar to the process of radio or television transmission. As a healer, you are able to shift your consciousness so that you can perceive the other person's four bodies. Like the TV set that acts as a relay or a reception box, with different channels coming through the airwaves, you as the healer perceive other energies. You correctly translate and sort them; you are able to feel what is going on with that person. You then send appropriate, supportive energy to help the person create his or her safe healing space.

One of my earlier cases in long distance healing occurred with a middle-aged female dog named Charlie. One evening, I was called at home by the frantic owner. Charlie was suffering a severe reaction to a flea medication. The vet had sent her home, unable to do anything else. A few days had gone by, but the animal showed no change and was listless, lying all day and night in her bed.

It was very early in my color healing career; I had no idea if it would even work, but I told the owner I would try. Around 10:00 pm, I began sending energy, focusing for about ten minutes. The next day, the owner called to say that Charlie had gotten up around 1:30 am, bouncing around the house like a puppy. From that point on, she showed no reaction to the flea medication, and was exceptionally exuberant.

One cannot be sure that my color healing helped this animal; however, the dog showed marked improvement shortly afterward. No doubt, much of the success of color healing with animals (and with plants) is their lack of mental resistance to it, unlike human beings.

Since that earlier time, I have participated in both single and group healings of a "long distance" nature. Without fail, people have reported very positive results back to us. However, if there were a choice, I would opt for hands-on healing rather than long distance work; close contact seems to be key to the healing process, especially for those who need to *feel* or *see* something. Long distance work can be intangible for many people. But, it is definitely possible and desirable when you can't physically be with someone.

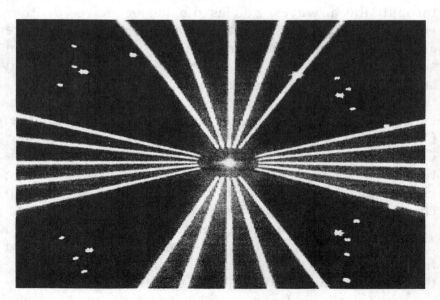

Chapter 12

Blocks, Balance, and the Ego

Blocks

From my point
of ultimate resistance

I move to a space
of complete peace.

I am Light, I am Love.
I am energy, I am movement.

I create from resistance
13 rays of perfect balance.

---Omega
8-26-91

As I mentioned in Chapter 8 all of our chakras are subject to our issues and our traumas which can create blockages. Any barriers within our energy systems keep us from experiencing the full expression of our gifts, ability to love others unconditionally, and divine illumination.

Bursting Through Blocks Technique

The following is an extremely effective technique for addressing the blockages at the cellular, physical, emotional, and mental levels. It will also align your spiritual essence with the previously mentioned bodies.

* Have the person lie down.
* Ask the four angels of north, south, east, and west to set the corners of the room.
* Ask for the White Brotherhood symbol (the magenta circle with the white cross within it) to envelop the room, so that everyone is protected, cared for, and guided.
* State to the person's physical body that its intent is to remove all blocks (such as blocks to physical healing, etc.). Ask whether or not that intent is acceptable. Have the person answer verbally.
* Next, address the emotional body: "We understand that in this particular essence there has been trauma and pain. But in this lifetime those are no longer needed. Now is the time to bring forth the wisdom of those lifetimes without the trauma and pain. Our intent is to clear the trauma and pain. Is this acceptable to the emotional body? Please answer aloud."
* Next, address the mental body: "Whatever data that has been brought forward, which is no longer perti-

nent, will be transmuted and put into alignment with your intent--only that data that is pertinent will now be brought forward. Is this an agreeable intent by the mental body? Please answer aloud."

- Now address the spiritual body: "All things are perfect and complete. The spiritual body is to be connected to these other 3 bodies in such a way that it brings light, movement, understanding, and wisdom. *It is the blueprint.* We would ask that at the level of the blueprint, anything that needs to be corrected, aligned, or enhanced be changed at this time. This is to be done for the highest level of intent, the highest good, and with alignment of free will. Does the spiritual body agree with this intent?"

- Now begin with the base chakra, one hand below, one hand above, both touching the body. Say: "In the Light of the Source, by the power vested in me as a healer, I would ask now that the physical body release any blocks to healing at this time, at whatever level is necessary." Encourage the blocks to let go, envision them spiraling upward and being transmuted.

- When the blocks are gone, ask the emotional body to release any blocks associated with that chakra.

- Ask or tell the mental body to release any data not in alignment with stated intent.

- State: "And now the spiritual body will tap into the Universe, the Creation, the Source, and from It will flow the 13 rays. These rays will flow into this chakra, harmonizing and balancing it at all levels, filling it with completion."

  NOTE: You never leave a void when a block is taken or dispersed. You always refill and balance.

- Swap hands for the next chakra (if the left hand was on bottom for base, it's now on top, etc.).

117

- Follow the same procedure at every chakra through the 3rd eye. Keep restating instructions and intent. "Release that which is no longer needed. Go to the RNA/DNA cellular level* if necessary."
- State: "In alignment with free will, I ask that this energy point release. Look at the mental body data that you bring forth to this essence, that which is *of* and which *supports* the highest good, and that which supports the *intent* of each chakra. You are whole and complete, you are abundant and perfect, you are aligned as a being of light, as a guardian of the universe."
- At the end of clearing the physical, emotional, and mental bodies at the third eye, switch the bottom hand to crown chakra, and leave the top hand on the third eye.
- Then say, "The 13 rays of creation will flow through this body at a complete cellular level, and will flow into the physical body, touching the physical body, and allowing the physical body to become a living rainbow. These rays will touch, bless, and link in such a way that this body radiates only perfect, abundant health."

---

* Some of the energy patterns within the body are housed within the RNA/DNA cellular coding handed down to us by our ancestors. To clear these patterns means to clear possible disease tendencies within our bodies.

Transmitting Color to Balance the Chakras

The purpose of this exercise is to transmute negative or inharmonious energy in the body's chakra system.

- Sit cross-legged on the floor, facing each other. Greet each other verbally or telepathically, "From the God of my being to the God of your being, I greet you in Light, Love, harmony, and balance."
- Determine which is the receiving hand and which is the transmitting hand. If you can use either hand for receiving/transmitting, pick whichever one you wish.
- Have the other person place his receiving hand on your transmitting hand. Take your receiving hand and place it above his or her crown chakra. Receive the *amethyst* shade of violet into your hand chakra. At the same time, bring the amethyst ray of your own crown chakra into your transmitting hand.
- Place your receiving hand on the earth. Send back into the earth an *emerald green* ball in which you've wrapped anything that your hand picked up that was misaligned, inharmonious, or imbalanced. (The emerald green comes from within your being and goes out accordingly.)
- Go to the next chakra (at the brow), receive and transmit that color (*indigo*), then follow with the hand on the earth as before.
- Transmit each chakra color in this manner, sequentially.

A variation of this technique is to have both participants transmit at the same time. If you are simply balancing one another, you can do it simultaneously. *If one of you has an illness, then you should __not__ simultaneously transmit energy. Illness can create an imbalance in your*

119

*energies; it would do neither participant any good to run
energy if one of you is sick.*

The Role of Ego in Healing

What place does ego have in the process of facilitating
healing for others? One would think that it has <u>no place</u>;
that expressing ego corrupts the clarity of the channeling.

That's not precisely true.

To understand the role of *ego* in the healing process, we
must first define the word by its original meaning.

Ego is the recognition of Self, at all the levels of being.
Without ego, you wouldn't have the ability to know who
you are. Without ego, there isn't personality, or the balanced energy of the soul. Ego is directly linked to the
process of sentience, the awareness of one's self as an in-
telligent essence.

What people refer to as an "ego trip" is actually an imbalance of the ego energy. It is what we call *alter ego*, or
what Webster's defines as someone's "other self." [It is
the misalignment of ego. Being excessively humble and
self-effacing is also alter ego -- "alter" means "to change."]
Alter ego encompasses ego dysfunctions, which often become learning lessons.

Ego is like the balance of the yin-yang energies. It is neither too far in the direction of the passive yin, nor too
close to the active yang.

The alter ego is in play when there is either too much
yin or yang. When the alter ego is consistently in the passive side, one is self-effacing and hasn't a true recognition
of his or her gifts and talents. When someone is consistently caught up in the active side, he or she has an
overly-important, superior view of self.

Most of my students initially seem to fall in the passive category. They are learning to appreciate their abilities, and are striving to become self-empowered and balanced in the yin-yang energies.

It is rare to find a completely balanced person. That is the challenge. We may approach middle ground from one side or another, then swing to the opposite end of the spectrum. It is an intense, often circuitous path to a balanced ego.

Ways to regain ego balance include: extensive work towards balancing the male/female energy within us, and clearing all our bodies: physical, emotional, mental, while aligning our spiritual body within these bodies, as well as remembering the many lifetimes of healing service we have already given. This self-acknowledgment will give you added confidence in your abilities, along with a greater understanding of how multifaceted and multi-talented you really are.

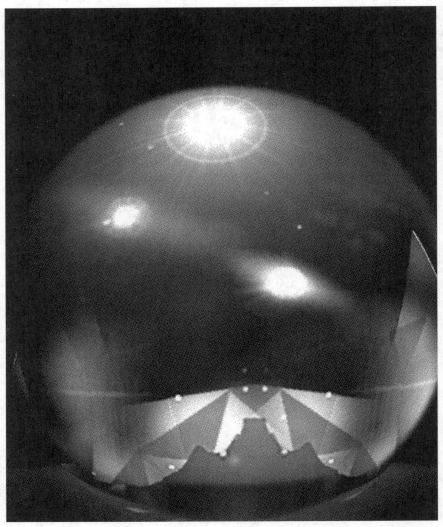

John Mason

Chapter 13

Causal Plane Connecting

Void

Space, time lost
Space, time found

Linking the void
to the soul.

Losing the part
finding the all.

---Voltra
8-26-91

The Buddha said, "We are what we think. All that we are arises with our thoughts. With our thoughts we make the world." We can have our thoughts reflect our divine perfection, or express a more limiting perspective. All that has ever been thought of permeates Creation (the macrocosm) and our view of reality (the microcosm). A record of all thought and action is kept within what is commonly known as the Akashic records, or the cosmic library. We, as individuals, have the option of embracing whatever thought patterns we desire. We constantly create and reinforce our reality at this physical level. At a subtle level we also create. This state of consciousness is called the **causal plane**.

The causal plane is cosmic Mind. A non-physical "place", it is where you create all of your simultaneous aspects or lifetimes. It is different from your mental body because it is apart from the time/space continuum we call linear time. Your mental body exists only in your current physical body.

You can visualize cosmic Mind, or the causal plane, in any form. Some people create a crystal world, a meadow, or an ocean shore. The important thing is that you feel comfortable in your special place.

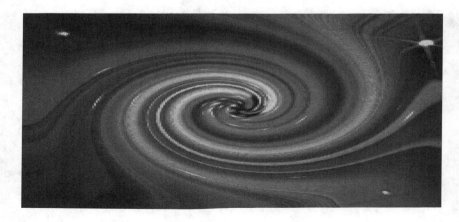

124

Moving Within the Causal Plane

- Lie or sit in a comfortable position.
- Visualize or feel each of your seven chakras. Bring the *violet* ray down through your crown chakra to the base chakra.
- Starting at the base chakra, replace the red with violet until you feel a shift in this area. The red is completely gone, replaced by violet energy.
- Repeat this with the spleen chakra, replacing the orange with violet.
- Do this with each chakra until you reach the crown. Add violet also to your crown chakra.
- At the crown chakra, you will feel or see a shape that is like a violet tornado. Allow yourself to enter the exterior flow of the storm and circle with it.
- After a few moments, leave the exterior and move into the eye of the tornado. *This is the causal plane.* There is no time or space. From this point, you may clear or create all you wish.

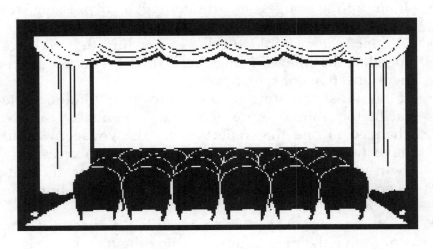

Causal Plane Clearing

When you are first starting out clearing within the causal plane is best done with a facilitator. A trained facilitator can ask pertinent questions that will trigger clearing, while supporting you through the process. I understand that some of you will not have a trained facilitator. In that case, work with someone you trust, preferably someone with an understanding of the healing arts. Connect with a local healing center; they should be able to assist you with valuable recommendations.

This process is done from the facilitator's perspective:

- The participant is in the causal plane awaiting your direction.
- Have the participant passively watch the screen in his mind, noting any images or movies that might appear.
- As the person begins to perceive images, see if they are "present or past" life experiences.
- If any of the images are frightening or depressing, remind him/her to remain detached.
- The facilitator should use his or her intuition to piece together the images being seen. It helps to ask pertinent questions of the voyager.
- If it is a disappointing or traumatic "past" lifetime, the facilitator should state that the experience can be changed to one that reflects what the voyager would have wanted it to be. What one wants to create is a "win-win" scenario, resisting retaliation or the get-even approach with someone who may have hurt the person.
- As the scenes unfold in a modified version of the story, give the person time to enjoy the new scenario.

- When finished, direct the person to bring the changed experience back with him/her, along with the positive feelings that go with it.
- Lead the voyager back into the eye of the vortex, then down into the crown chakra. Change the crown back to the normal shade and amount of violet.
- Next, go to the third eye and change it back to indigo. Proceed through each chakra the same way, adjusting each until it returns to its usual and original color.

Causal Plane Creation

In a sense, when you *clear* a past life circumstance to reflect a better scenario, you also *create*. In fact, you can go to the causal plane specifically to create or manifest positive situations in your life. One way to do this is as follows:

- Lead the person into the causal plane.
- The facilitator then asks the voyager to erect a blank screen in his/her mind.
- The voyager creates upon this internal screen of what he/she wishes to manifest in life. It can be anything that the voyager desires, be it a better job, a relationship, spiritual progress, etc..
- Blocks to expression or manifestation can be obliterated when creative energy is focused at causal level. Have the voyager see where the blockages are, then watch as the blocks dissolve in his/her mind's eye.
- When finished, direct the person to bring the manifestation back with him/her.
- Lead the voyager back into the eye of the vortex, then down into the crown chakra. Change the crown back to the normal shade and amount of violet.

- Next, go to the third eye and change it back to indigo. Proceed through each chakra the same way as described in the previous exercise.

This causal plane technique is one of the most powerful I have worked with. It accesses very deep-seated problems. A participant expressed to me (after only one session), "I feel like a heavy weight that has always been on me has gone away." Others have been able to rid themselves of destructive patterns, or have been able to manifest specific things they want in life; such as increasing harmony with interpersonal relationships, obtaining a meaningful career, or developing a spiritual ability.

If you are facilitating another person for purposes of clearing, be aware that the client may become quite emotional by the internally driven pictures he or she is viewing. If this happens, it is advisable to repeatedly remind the voyager to detach or step back. Frequently, the client may be caught up in a past life experience, reliving too intensely a past life trauma such as injury or death. Remind them gently but firmly that they are "only an observer."

It is O.K. to do this technique by yourself, but I recommend that you do this only after being facilitated during your first attempt by someone trained in the technique. Initially, work with the manifestation process and save any major past or present life clearings until you can work with someone you trust.

What would happen if you went into a spontaneous clearing while in the causal plane? You would simply fall asleep. At that level, the Higher Self would spare you from going through something you would be unable to handle alone.

Looking at Your Own Cellular Structure

Purpose: To understand how your own physiology functions.

- Sit in a cross-legged position, or in a comfortable chair. Place a lighted candle in front of you.

- Find a fixed point of light within the flame of the candle. Follow your breathing for approximately 5--10 minutes.

- Move your consciousness from the body, projecting into the flame of the candle so you are viewing the body from the outside.

- Gaze into the candle for 15--30 minutes until you are a part of it, and until you no longer feel the physical body. Breathe naturally.

- Now *look* with your psychic eyes into your body to see the heart, circulatory system, the nervous system, etc. (Remember, use your strongest psychic ability: hearing, seeing, feeling or knowing.)

- When you are completed, gently return your consciousness back into the physical body.

- Ground yourself.

NOTE: In this altered state you have the capability of changing your blood pressure and altering the physiology of your body. You'd be able to take a pin, touch it to any part of your body without a response. This altered state allows you to control what has always been termed *autonomic* physiological responses of the body, that which operates independently of will under the control of the central nervous system. *This altered state is part of the process that occurs during psychic healing or psychic surgery.*

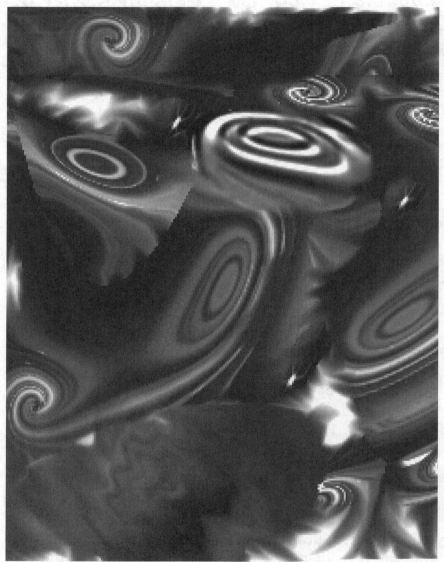

Sarah Steinbach

Chapter 14

Blending, Merging, and Ley Line Connecting

Universal Grids

Webs of creation
Lights ever commingling

Vortices of realization
spirals ever spinning

Wheels within wheels
circling for time immemorial

---Korton
8-26-91

During the early history of Earth, people understood how to work with the energies and the cycles of life. They knew that some aspects of life were physical, some were emotional, others were mental, and that some of life's aspects were spiritual. Everything had a natural cycle to it; the people functioned from a holographic or a spiraling point of view. As humanity became more linear in their thinking processes, they lost the ability to function within natural cycles, and to understand those cycles.

The purpose of the next three techniques is to teach you how to reconnect with all parts of yourself, to re-address yourself as a holographic being. This will be in opposition to the linear-style separateness you have become used to.

Blending Rays

- Work with a partner. Sit opposite one another, about a foot apart. Choose who will go first. (At the end of the technique you can switch roles.)
- Place one hand at the crown chakra, the other at the base chakra. Pull the rays *violet* and *red* together combining them at the heart chakra. This creates the blended color of **magenta**, which signifies "protection."
- Dissipate the energy before going to the next step. To do this, just imagine the energy as dissolving away as you stop the flow.
- Repeat the same process, placing one hand at the third eye and the other at the spleen. Pull the *indigo* and *orange* rays into the heart. **Sienna** is the blend of these two rays. This color signifies the "reproductive energy of the earth" and "clarity through creation."
- Dissipate the energy before going to the next step.

Repeat the process, bringing *translucent blue* and *yellow* into the heart. **Sea-foam green** is the blended color that will be created. It signifies "rebirth, renewal, cleansing of the emotions and spirit."

- Dissipate the energy before going to the next step.
- Place both hands at the heart, drawing together the *rose* and *green* rays. Combined, they make up the aspects of the **clear** ray.* Each primary pigment is present: red, yellow, blue. This signifies "balance at all levels."
- Dissipate the energy. Clear and ground yourself.

Aura Merging

The purpose of this technique is to delve a little deeper into these powerful blended energies by temporarily merging your auric field with your partner's.

- Sit with a partner. Face each other. Determine who will transmit and who will receive.
- The transmitter brings the *red* ray from the base chakra up to the heart chakra and simultaneously brings the *violet* ray from the crown chakra down to the heart. As they blend at the heart the radiant color created is **magenta**.
- Send this magenta color into your partner's heart. Feel it expand and encompass both of your auras in a large bubble.
- Let the energy dissipate before you run the next colors.
- The transmitter then brings the *orange* of the spleen chakra up to the heart and simultaneously brings the

---

* Why do the rose and green rays blend into the clear ray, rather than the white ray or another color? The physical body is expressed by the green ray and the emotional body by the rose ray. Most of the human confusion occurs at the physical and emotional levels. When the two combine in this manner, they create *clarity* or the understanding of the clear ray. Although every primary pigment is present, it is really not about pigment, but about radiant color.

133

third eye *indigo* color down to the heart. The blended radiant color is **sienna**.

- Send this energy into your partner's heart. Let it expand to encompass both of your auras in a large bubble.
- Let the energy disburse before you run the next colors.
- The transmitter then brings the *yellow* from the solar plexus to the heart chakra and simultaneously brings the *translucent blue* from the throat chakra to the heart. The blended color is **seafoam green**.
- Send this energy into the heart of your partner, letting it expand to encompass both of you in a large bubble.
- Let the energy disburse before you run the next colors.
- The transmitter then brings the partner's *rose* and *green* energies (at the heart chakra) together. The resulting radiant color is the **clear** ray. Let this blended energy expand to encompass your auras.
- Let the energy disburse. Ground and clear.

Ley Line Tying

The Earth contains many magnetic anomalies. Some of these are called "mystery spots" where modern instrumentation fluctuates wildly. Pilots avoid flying in those areas, for obvious reasons.

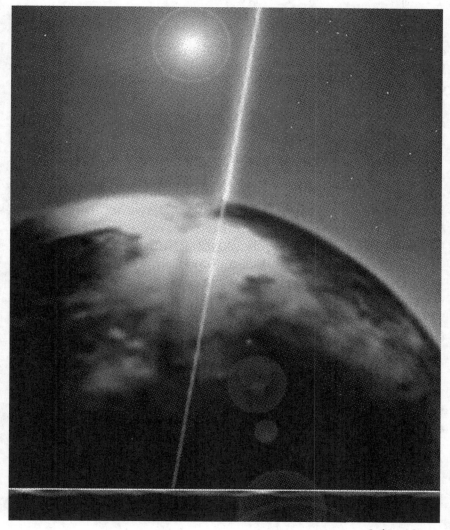

John Mason

With a process called Kirlian photography, we are now able to photograph Earth's auric field. These photos clearly show energy grids and patterns. By photographing Earth with ultraviolet or infrared spectrum lighting we can capture the varying heat and light on film. Combined, these techniques help to define the magnetic resonance of the Earth. The planet's energies come together as *ley lines*.

Ley lines are electromagnetic; they crisscross the earth and are connected to certain vortices, or concentrations of energy. Within these vortices all energy is amplified, whether it be positive or negative. Psychic abilities are enhanced at these charged points; energy is expanded and healing takes place. Much like the human body's chakra system, the planet Earth has a chakra system, as well.

Ley lines connect us to the planet. In doing so we connect to the feminine energy and the balanced yin-yang. This facilitates the process of correcting any imbalance in ourselves.

Non-physical ley lines also exist. Many people in the metaphysical field have not delved into them. While our ability to perceive non-physical ley lines is more subtle, they are quite powerful. (Soul essences in human bodies also have non-physical chakras.)

This ley line tying technique will acquaint you with the various physical and non-physical ley lines. The function of this exercise is not to offer detailed specifics of each ley line, merely to acknowledge their existence. As with most of the techniques in this book, there is additional work that can be done. Greater depth and intensity of such energy work is best done in a one-on-one tutoring situation or in a classroom environment.

• Sit comfortably. Protect the body with white light. (To do so, merely visualize your auric field as being completely surrounded in a white cocoon of light.)

- Send *silver* energy into the Earth's core, connecting you to a point in the planet's center.
- Send *gold* energy to the center of the Creator. Connect to the center of Spirit.
- Bring *red* from the base chakra up to the heart and *violet* from the crown chakra down to the heart. At the heart chakra, combine the two rays to make *magenta*. Project the energy out from the heart and connect it to the **protective ley line** within the non-physical grid surrounding the Earth. (Don't be concerned <u>where</u> it is located; by asking for it with intent, the connection will automatically be made.) After a few minutes, disconnect by dissipating the energy link.
- Bring the *orange* ray from the spleen chakra up to the heart chakra and bring the *indigo* ray from the 3rd eye down to the heart. Combined, the radiant color created is *sienna*. Project the blended color out from the heart chakra and connect with the **clarity/creative ley line** within the non-physical grid surrounding the planet. Dissipate the link before going on to the next connection.
- Bring the *yellow* ray up from the solar plexus to the heart chakra and bring the *translucent blue* from the throat down to the heart. The radiant color created is *sea-foam green.*. Project the blended rays out from the heart center and connect with the **rebirth, renewal, emotional/spiritual cleansing ley line** within the non-physical grid surrounding the Earth. Dissipate the link when complete.
- At the heart chakra, bring the *rose* and *green* rays forth to create the *clear* ray. Project the blended rays out from the heart chakra and connect with the **male/female ley line** within the non-physical grid surrounding the planet. Dissipate the link when complete.

- At this point, bring forth the *red* ray from the base chakra and project it out to connect with the **physical, grounding ley line** within the physical Earth grid. Dissipate the link when complete.
- Next, project the *orange* ray from the spleen chakra and connect it to the **sexual energy ley line** within the physical Earth grid. Dissipate the link when complete.
- Project the *yellow* ray from the solar plexus chakra and connect it to the **power ley line** within the physical Earth grid. Dissipate the link when complete.
- Now, project the *green* ray from the heart chakra and connect it to the **healing ley line** within the physical Earth grid. Dissipate the link when complete.
- Connect the *rose* ray from the heart chakra to the **love ley line** within the physical Earth grid. Dissipate the link when complete.
- Next, connect the *translucent blue* ray from the throat chakra to the **communication ley line** within the physical Earth grid. Dissipate the link when complete.
- Connect the *indigo* from the third eye to the **psychic sight, spiritual ley line** within the physical Earth grid. Dissipate the link when complete.
- Finally, connect the *purple* of the crown chakra to the **wisdom ley line** within the physical Earth grid. Dissipate the link when complete.
- Clear completely and then ground.

Each person's experience of these ley lines will be unique. Some may feel more connected to the physical ley lines; others will relate more to the non-physical ley lines, or only to certain ones, physical or non-physical. Perceptions will vary widely; many will have profound psychic experiences, others will just sense a nice energy while connected to the ley lines.

Connecting with the Four Bodies of Earth

This is a wonderful technique you can use to connect in an intimate way with Mother Earth. Afterwards, you will have a clearer understanding of the four primary aspects of the living Earth. You will realize that she is as alive as we are. You will be able to provide wonderful healing energy by **grounding** the spiritual rays of light into these aspects.

- Sit on the ground with a group of people in a circle. Hold hands. (If you are alone, place your hands on the ground next to you.)
- Take a few deep, cleansing breaths. Feel the Earth physically.
- Expand your aura, out from your body, to where you psychically sense the Earth's **physical** body. Use the *black* ray to become part of the Earth's "physicalness."
- Now expand your aura using the *rose* ray. Move into the **emotional** body of Earth.
- Expand your aura farther out until you touch the **mental** body of Earth. Use the *white* ray to do this.
- Now touch the **spiritual** body using the *clear* ray.

  The clear ray is the "pure intent of Earth." It surrounds the group.

- Ask the spirit of the Earth, whose name is *Gaia* (pronounced Gay-e-a): "In the Light and Love of the Source, Gaia, would you share your **spiritual intent** with us?"
- As you tune in to what she is saying, you may state it verbally. [This process is called *channeling*, which was explained in Chapter 4.]

139

- When this is completed, state "In the Light and Love of the Source, Gaia, would you share your **mental data** with us?"
- As you receive answers, you may verbally express them with the group.
- "In the Light and Love of the Source, Gaia, would you share your **emotional expression** with us?"
- As you tune in to what she is saying, you may state it orally.
- "In the Light and Love of the Source, Gaia, what would you manifest **physically**?"
- As you receive answers, you may share them with the group verbally.
- Ask now for all 13 rays of color to be present. Create a rainbow of the following rays:

Red

Orange

Yellow

Green

Rose

Translucent Blue

Indigo

Violet

Silver

Gold

White

Clear

Black

- Have the rainbow of the 13 rays spiral out and surround the whole Earth--the Earth itself, along with the various beings that inhabit it, will draw whatever color they need from this rainbow.
- Allow the energy to slowly disburse.
- Clear!

- At this time, walk down from Spirit. To do this, start with the *clear* ray. Dissipate the clear ray energy connection to the spiritual body of Earth.
- Feel the *white* ray, disburse the white ray energy connection to the mental body of Earth.
- Tune into the *rose* ray. Dissipate the rose ray energy connection to the emotional body of Earth.
- Use the *black* ray to balance to the physical Earth. Allow the excess black ray energy dissipate into the Earth.

The Mystical Healing Space

Throughout history, many different philosophers, spiritual, and mystical people have spoken about a sacred space that exists within each person; a place that represents the soul. Within that soul is the connection between the physical world and one's link to the Eternal Presence. It is believed by ancient cultures that the Earth also has a soul. Within the soul of the Earth, that sacred space is called the Halls of Amente. It contains the recorded history of Earth's soul, and is located underground. There is a similar sacred space within all celestial bodies, such as a planet, sun, or galaxy. When you are in tune with your own soul essence, you have the ability to journey within the soul essence of such sacred bodies. From the point that exists outside of time and space, you gain knowledge. It is not only beneficial for you, but beneficial for the rest of Creation.

With the destruction of Atlantis, Lemuria, and Sumeria (the ancient "lost" civilizations of the Earth), and the shifting of the three main continents of the Earth, the spiritual centers **Shangri-La, Shambhala, Montecillio** still existed at the higher dimensional levels. These spiritual "cities" were blueprints for ancient civilizations.

Shambhala was the spiritual city for Atlantis, Shangri-La was the spiritual city for Sumeria, and Montecillio was the sister city of Lemuria. They were commonly thought to be floating above Earth in a highly refined dimensional space, or overlaid over the original locations.

Today, the planet is re-linking these three centers and the Halls of Amente, for the purpose of healing, and to connect Earth to other-dimensional states of consciousness. The following exercise will allow you to become part of this sacred re-linking process.

Time vaults are power spots upon the Earth where the ancients stored important, advanced data before the collapse of their civilizations. This data cannot be activated until the mass consciousness of the people on this planet has evolved into a much more enlightened state. However, one can tap into the spiritual energy of the vaults.

This is to be done in a large group (a minimum of 13 people). There should be 4 facilitators, placed at each corner, just outside the circle.

- Form a circle. Position 3 people in the center of the circle. (They will represent the *clear*, *white*, and *black* rays, acting as anchors to hold the energy.)
- Each of the other participants will represent a color ray. The rays begin with *red* represented at the south end of the circle, successive colors are represented in a counter-clockwise order, ending with *gold*. If there are more people, just begin the color sequence again. (See Chart. 14-1)
- The three persons representing the clear, white, and black rays will send energy to each person in the outer circle.
- Persons representing the other colors will also send their specific color ray energy back into the middle of the circle to form a triad. This creates a rainbow effect.
- The energy should build and build, literally producing a space of pure Creation energy.

- Spiritually link into the time vault at Mt. Shasta to link with the Lemurian energy, the extraterrestrial energy, and the White Brotherhood energy.
- Next, send the energy to all of the other vaults on the planet. (See Chart 14-2)

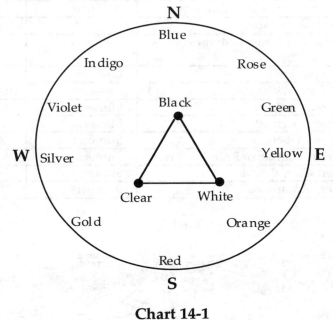

Chart 14-1

- Then, direct that energy to spread itself to the three spiritual cities (Shambhala, Shangri-La, Montecillio) to form a triad. This will take you through all the Earth's dimensions, linking you to the Higher Self of the Earth (Gaia).
- Now, take the energy and funnel it back down the dimensional layers of the planet deep into the Earth, to the Halls of Amente.
- Upon completion, be sure to allow the energy to dissipate. Ground and clear!

Time Vaults

Time Vault	Culture	Ray
Great Zimbabwe, Africa	Atlantis	Red
Thebes--Sacred Lake, Egypt	Atlantis	Orange
Pyramid of Cheops at Ghiza, Egypt	Atlantis	Yellow
Chichen Itza, Yucatan	Lemuria	Green
Mt. Shasta, California/ Montezuma's Castle, Arizona	Lemuria	Rose
Machu Pichu, Peru	Lemuria	Blue
Grand Tetons, Wyoming	Lemuria	Indigo
Mt. Arrarat, Turkey	Sumeria	Violet
Stonehenge, England	Sumeria	Silver
Mt. Everest, Tibet	Sumeria	Gold
Isle of Crete, Temple of Knossos, Greece	Sumeria	White
Forbidden City, China	Sumeria	Clear
Mt. Sister, Antarctica	Atlantis	Black

Chart 14-2

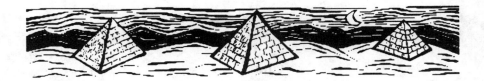

Chapter 15

Color, Sound, and Movement

Myriads of Motion

Myriads of motion
Prisms everyone

Dancing to a memory
Moving to serenity

Hearing every prism
Feeling every sound

---Elycia
July 1991

Meanings of the Colors at Your Chakras

Very few people have as their chakra colors the primary or standard shades of each color. We vary in our expressions; the multiple shades of color reflect those variations. Each shade or frequency has its own meaning, and it tells a story about us.

For this exercise, you will need to obtain a box of color crayons. I have used the Crayola® brand. Separate the shades, as listed, into separate piles or containers. For each of your chakras, pick the color with which you most closely resonate. There may be more than one color that fits you; conversely, no singular color may feel quite right. In that case, you will have to mix two or more colors together to create a blended energy. I recommend that you mix blended colors on a separate sheet of paper in order to avoid confusion. For your final selections, write down the names of each color or set of blended colors. *Do not look at the color shade meanings until you have selected your color(s); it may bias you in your selection.*

You may use Chart 15-1 to color the chakras with your selected shades.

The meanings of the color shades are covered in the following pages.

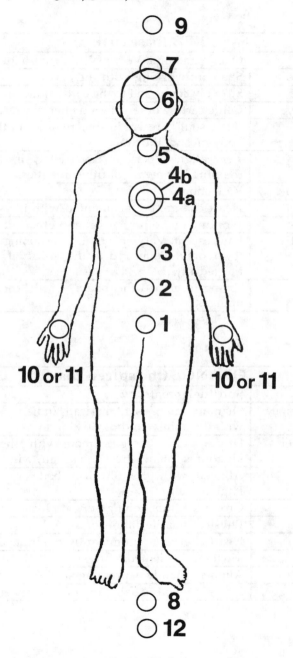

Chart 15-1

RED (base chakra)	
Copper	Open kundalini. Very psychic, runs a lot of energy
Indian Red	Shaman; working with the earth
Sepia	Strongly connected to the earth; quite grounded
Mahogany	Celtic earth workers; Druid energy workers
Brick Red	"New soul". Present in this reality. In the physical body most of the time.
Red	Very aligned person. Completely in the body all the time but aware of other realities.
Maroon	Protection
Red Violet	Heart chakra; not acquainted with physical body
Violet Red	Working on both physical and other planes; aligned
Ultra Red	Fluorescent. Very spiritual. Functioning on spiritual level only. Connected to the spiritual guardian of the red ray.
Tan	Trying to ground the body. Earth combined with orange.

ORANGE (the spleen chakra)	
Apricot	Spiritual creativity
Burnt Orange	Shaman energies; American Indian. Works more with the animal and devic kingdoms
Bittersweet	Druid, Celtic energies; more with the elemental kingdoms (plants, trees, rocks, air, wind, water)
Orange	Aligned with the physical body as well as the Higher Self
Red Orange	Grounded; functioning only at physical level
Orange Red	Physical manifestation only
Melon	Heart chakra, predominantly feminine energy
Yellow Orange	Movement oriented; powerful in their energy
Peach	Aligned; mainly expressing spiritual body
Ultra Orange	Not in the body at all; pure orange ray energy

YELLOW (the solar plexus chakra)	
Goldenrod	Grounded
Maize	Shaman
Lemon Yellow	Druid energy
Yellow Yellow	Physical
Chartreuse	Green yellow. Heart energy coming through.
Orange Yellow	Expresses physically and creatively; artists
Gold	Masculine, aligned; spiritual expression through the physical body
Ultra Yellow	Translucent; often out of the body

GREEN (the heart chakra--physical)	
Olive	Grounded
Pine Green	Shaman energy
Forest Green	Druid energy
Green Green	Physically present
Yellow Green Green Yellow	Expresses through solar plexus; power center
Sea Green	Expresses through heart chakra
Spring Green	Expresses spirit
Ultra Green	Similar to emerald; spiritual functioning only

ROSE (the heart chakra--emotional)	
Magenta	Grounded; protective
Hot Magenta	Very physical; grounds and protects
Salmon	Indian shaman
Thistle	Druid energy
Carnation Pink	Predominantly emotional body. Moving from heart chakra, unconditional love
Ultra Pink	Spiritual love; translucent

TRANSLUCENT BLUE (the throat chakra)	
Blue Gray	Grounded (because of the black pigment within the color)
Turquoise Blue	Shaman energy
Green Blue Blue Green	Druid energy
Aquamarine	Aligned physically; expressing through throat energy
Sky Blue	Communicator through heart chakra, emotional body
Periwinkle	Expressing through heart chakra; counseling strengths
Cadet Blue	Expressing through mental body

INDIGO (the third eye chakra)	
Midnight Blue	Contains black energy; grounded
Cornflower	Shaman energy
Violet Blue	Druid energy
Navy Blue	Dealing with the mental body
Blue	Mental body and communication. Combines third eye and throat chakras
Ultra Blue	An open 3rd eye; psychic.

VIOLET (the crown chakra)	
Mulberry	Grounded
Orchid	Druid
Blue Violet	Mental body expression
Lavender	Emotional body expression
Violet	True crown energy. Spiritual expression
Plum	Shaman
Silver	Feminine energy
Gold	Masculine energy
White	Spiritual protection is the focus
Clear	The focus is spiritual truth
Black	Movement; the energy of testing oneself

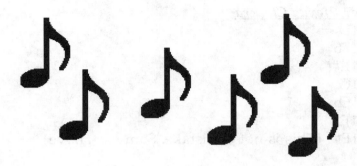

Your Personal Sound

From each chakra group select a note with which you intuitively resonate. See Fig. 15.2 for keyboard location of notes.

Base Chakra:
-2Db (Two octaves below middle C)
-2D#
-2C
-2D
-2Fb
-2F
-2F#

Spleen Chakra:
-2G
-2A
-1Cb
-1C (One octave below middle C)
-2G#
-2A#
-1C#

Solar Plexus Chakra
    -1D
    -1Fb
    -1E#
    -1G
    -1Eb
    -1F#
    -1F#   (This is not a mistake. Same as above)

Heart Chakra

Green aspect	Rose aspect
-1A	Middle Cb
Middle Cb	Middle C
Middle C	Middle D
Middle D	Middle Fb
-1B	Middle C#
Middle Db	Middle D#
Middle C#	Middle D# (Same as above)

Throat Chakra
    Middle E
    Middle E#
    Middle G
    Middle A
    Middle Eb
    Middle F#
    Middle Ab

Third Eye
Middle A
Middle B
+1C (One octave above middle C)
+1E
Middle Bb
+1C#
+1Db

Crown Chakra
+1D
+1E
+1F
+1G
+1A
+1F#
+1Ab

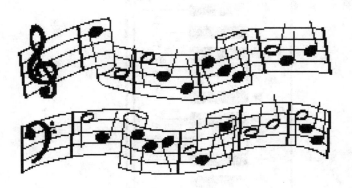

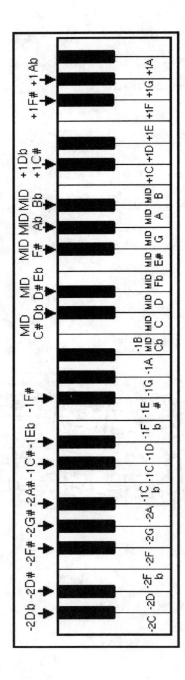

Fig. 15.2

What Do The Notes Mean?

Sharps (#) are feminine.
Flats (b) are masculine.
White keys (neither sharp nor flat) are androgynous.

- Notice which of your chakras have a feminine expression.
- Notice which of your chakras have a masculine expression.
- Notice which of your chakras have both aspects.
- When you have selected them all, play the notes (in order) from the base chakra to the crown chakra. It will be your musical signature.

There is a pattern to all of this:

The **base** chakra has predominantly male or balanced energy. At this deeper, more physical level you need more movement (which the male energy provides).

The **spleen** chakra is predominantly female or balanced energy. At this level there is creativity, the holding of the child at a physical level. (Even the creative male sperm is held at this level.) It is this way for the protection of the human race.

The **solar plexus** chakra is predominantly female or balanced energy. In the ancient Druid and shamanistic cultures, it was always the feminine aspect that held the energy for the male so he could move outward. What is created at our solar plexus is a mini-womb of energy.

The **green heart** chakra at the physical level is primarily balanced or androgynous energy. There is an extra note of the male energy; this provides movement.

The **rose heart** chakra at the emotional level is primarily female and balanced energy. The female carries more of the emotional or fluid energies.

The **throat** chakra is balanced between the combined male/female energies. There is an equal number of male and female notes. This aids communication.

The **third eye** is predominantly male, with the other notes being androgynous. If you think about it, the third eye is usually thought of as having mystical or psychic (balanced energy) or the left-brained, logic (male energy).

The **crown** chakra is almost exclusively androgynous, with an additional one note being female, one note being male. The crown represents complete androgyny, wisdom, and wholeness.

Movements and Your Chakras

The practice of Tai Chi, Tae Kwon Do, or other energy movements facilitates the alignment of your four bodies through the medium of movement. They are wonderfully empowering practices. We, as individuals, come into this incarnation with our own personal set of movements. This allows us to balance our chakras, permitting our energies to flow without blockages.

Each chakra has four movements, one of which will be suited for your body. These chakra movements are vibrationally attuned to the chakra system of the physical body. All four of the movements are very beneficial; however, for each chakra you will resonate more with one than with the others. Look at the following photographs and select one for each chakra.

After you have selected them, look at the meanings. Balance yourself daily by doing each movement in order, from base chakra to crown, in a slow, flowing manner.

As a variation, you can do <u>all</u> the movements in order. This provides an intense energy alignment of the chakras.

Movement - Physical
Base-1

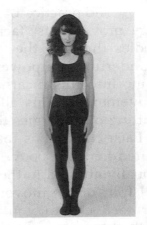

1A

Head tilted downward. Arms at sides. Legs together.

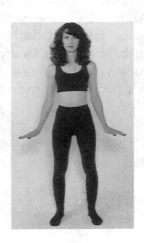

1B

Head forward. Arms at sides with palms down. Legs apart.

Movement - Physical
Base-1

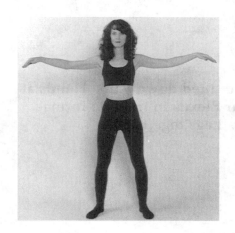

1C
Head forward. Arms out-stretched at sides. Palms down. Legs apart.

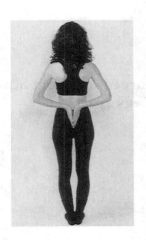

1D

<u>Back View</u>
Head tilted backward. Arms behind back, palms touching. Legs together

Movement - Physical
Spleen-2

2A

Head tilted downward. Hands at
Solar Plexus in triangle formation. Legs together.

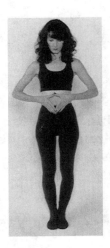

2B

Arms curved out front at waist
level. Legs apart.

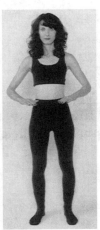

Movement - Physical
Spleen-2

<u>2C</u>

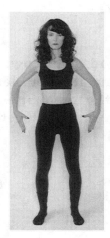

Arms curved at sides. Legs
apart.

<u>2D</u>

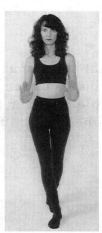

Hands out-stretched at waist
level. Right leg in front of left
leg about a foot distance.

Movement - Physical
<u>*Solar Plexus-3*</u>

<u>3A</u>

Head tilted downward. Right
hand at Solar Plexus palm up.
Left hand at Spleen Chakra, palm
down. Legs together.

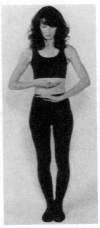

<u>3B</u>

Right leg bent at knee; right foot
against left knee. Left hand at solar plexus, palm up. Right arm
overhead, palm facing center.

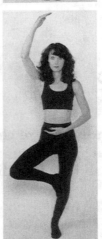

Movement - Physical
Solar Plexus-3

<u>3C</u>

Left hand at solar plexus, palm up. Right arm overhead, palm facing center. Right leg in front of left leg about a foot distance.

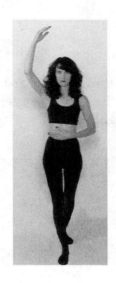

<u>3D</u>

Sit on floor. Left leg under buttocks. Right leg facing forward, knee bent with lower leg crossed over left leg. Arms at sides.

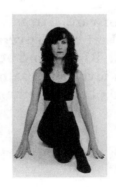

Movement - Emotional
Heart-Green-4

4A

Head tilted downward. Hands at Heart Chakra in prayer position. Legs together.

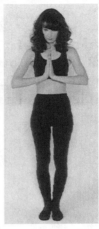

4B

Head forward. Arms bent at elbows. Left hand covers Heart Chakra. Right hand at Heart Chakra level with palm facing forward. Legs together.

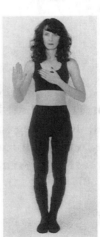

Movement - Emotional
Heart-Green-4

4C

Arms bent at elbows, left
hand covers Heart
Chakra. Right hand at
Heart Chakra level with,
palm up. Legs together.

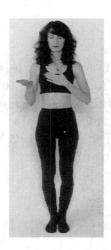

4D

Arms bent at elbows.
Hands out at Heart
Chakra level with,
palms up. Legs apart.

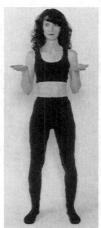

Movement - Emotional
Heart-Rose-4

4E

Arms bent at elbows, left hand
at Heart Chakra, palm toward
center. Right hand at Heart
Chakra level with palm up.
Right leg in front of left leg
about a foot distance.

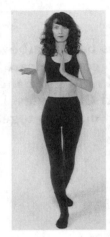

4F

Arms bent at elbows. Hands out
at Heart Chakra, palms up. Legs
together.

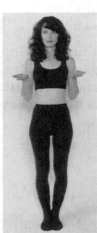

Movement - Emotional
Heart-Rose-4

4G

Hands at Heart Chakra in prayer
position. Right leg in front of
left leg, right heel touching toes
of left foot. Knees slightly bent.

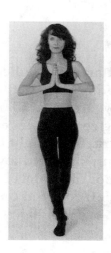

4H

Arms out at sides, elbows bent.
Legs apart. Knees bent.

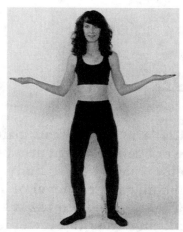

Movement - Emotional
Throat-5

5A

Right arm above head, palm
toward center. Left arm bent at
elbow, arm next to body, hand
facing center at level of Throat
Chakra. Bend right leg at knee,
placing knee and lower leg flat
on floor. Bend left leg at knee,
with left foot flat on floor.

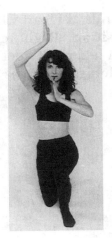

5B

Left arm above head, palm toward center. Right arm bent at
elbow, arm next to body, hand
facing center at level of Throat
Chakra. Bend left leg at knee,
placing knee and lower leg flat
on floor. Bend right leg at knee,
with right foot flat on floor.

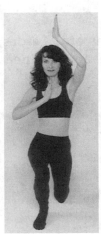

Movement - Emotional
Throat-5

<u>5C</u>

Sitting on floor, legs
crossed in "Lotus"
position. Arms rest-
ing at sides, palms
upturned on thighs.

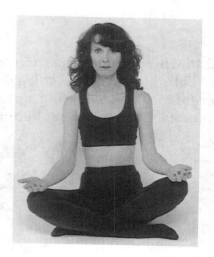

<u>5D</u>

Head touching floor, arms stretched out on floor above
head, palms down. Both legs bent at knees and tucked
under torso covering upper legs.

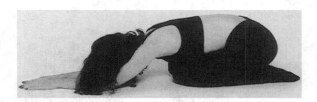

Movement - Mental/Spiritual
Third Eye-6

6A

Head touching floor, arms stretched out on floor above head. Palms down. Right leg bent at knee and tucked under torso. Torso covering upper leg. (Knee may touch chin.) Left leg stretched out behind.

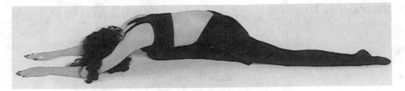

6B

Head touching floor, arms stretched out on floor above head. Palms up. Both legs bent at knees and tucked under torso. Torso covering upper legs.

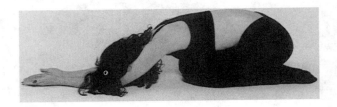

Movement - Mental/Spiritual
Third Eye-6

6C

Head touching floor, arms stretched out on floor above head. Palms down. Left leg bent at knee and tucked under torso. Torso covering upper leg. (Knee may touch chin.) Right leg stretched out behind.

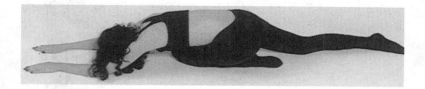

6D

Standing position. Arms above head, palms touching. Legs apart.

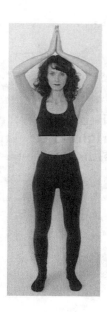

Movement - Mental/Spiritual
Crown-7

7A

Right leg bent at knee; right foot
against left knee. Arms above
head, palms together.

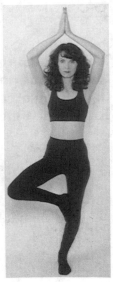

7B

Left leg bent at knee; left foot
against right knee. Arms above
head, palms together.

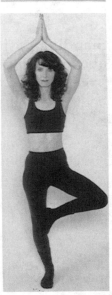

Movement - Mental/Spiritual
Crown-7

7C

Bend left leg at knee, placing knee and lower leg flat on the floor. Bend right leg at knee, with right foot flat on the floor. Arms overhead, palms together.

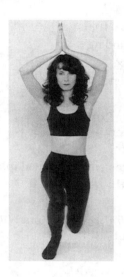

7D

Sit on floor with left leg under buttocks and right leg facing forward; knee bent with lower leg crossed under left leg. Arms overhead, palms together.

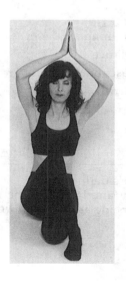

173

Meanings of Each Movement

First Chakra
1a	Stasis (balance)
1b	Grounding
1c	Peace
1c	Presence

Second Chakra
2a	Elemental
2b	Progressive
2c	Obelisk[1]
2d	Tao (void of creation)

Third Chakra
3a	Power
3b	Kinetic
3c	Terrestrial (physical planet)
3d	Earth

Fourth Chakra Physical (Green)
4a	Being
4b	Greet
4c	Acknowledge
4d	Exchange

Fourth Chakra Emotional (Rose)
4e	Feel
4f	Touch
4g	Connected
4h	At-oneness

Fifth Chakra
5a	Communicate
5b	Truth
5c	Cosmic
5d	Direction

Sixth Chakra
6a	Feminine
6b	Balance
6c	Masculine
6d	Spiral

Seventh Chakra
7a	Radiance
7b	Wholeness
7c	Starburst
7d	Totality

---

[1] Webster's defines *obelisk* as "A tall four-sided stone pillar taper-ing to its pyramidal top." The movement meaning here would indicate a person being as strong, powerful, and energy-directed as the obelisk.

Chapter 16

The Rays and the Origin of Creation

"*If God created the world, where was He before Creation? ... Know that the world is uncreated, as time itself is, without beginning and end.*"

---Mahapurana
(India, 9th century)

The Black Ray

At this time, I wish to discuss a much maligned color ray---the black ray.

What a "bad rap" the black ray has gotten for many centuries! It has been associated with black magic, voodoo, evil, and other forms of negativity. It seems that the only time black (as a color) is seen as attractive is in slimming clothing, leather jackets, cars, and modern decor.

Even many metaphysicians have not seen the black ray as a valid aspect of Light. It is frequently viewed as the flip side of white Light, lacking color, vibrancy, and the Creator's Touch. I've even heard some people say it's not really a color at all!

Where the black ray is concerned, true fear is shown by many. They fear what they don't understand. There is an old saying that the word *fear* really stands for *false evidence appearing real*.

The black ray is only energy, susceptible to use or misuse. Like any of the other color rays, the black ray can be used for unenlightened intent.

In the Star Wars movies, Darth Vador and Luke Skywalker both used "the Force." Skywalker used it in a non-manipulating positive manner. Vador used "the Force" to negatively control others and to gain power.

The black ray contains all of the other rays, as does the white ray and the clear ray. It comes directly from the Source, yet it always remains within It. The Source or Womb may look dark, or black, until one observes that It is really countless sparks of radiant color!

Aspects of the black ray leave the Womb and become guardians of the other color rays. These aspects are like different vibrational signatures of the black ray energy.[*]

---

[*] This will be further explained in Chapter 21.

When activated within these other color rays, the black energy provides movement, grounding, and testing.

Black, together with the clear ray (clarity, truth) and the white ray (protection), form a triad of energy comprising the spiritual blueprint of Creation. This blueprint embraces all of Creation, holding the representative colors of Creation, along with Its laws: Light, Love, Free Will, and Balance.

Throughout Creation's multiple dimensions, the black ray continues to play its role as mover and shaker. Its most intense work can be observed on physical dimensions where there is duality. At this time, the most concentrated duality can be found in the densest dimension of all--planet Earth.

My spiritual teachers state that Creation existed once before, then went back into the Source. Originally, when Creation came out of the Womb, the black ray was not a part of each ray. After a relatively short time, Creation imploded in on Itself, due to a lack of movement. The Source decided that for Creation to expand and evolve, the black ray was a needed key ingredient; it would prevent stagnation. A black ray guardian was placed within each rainbow ray.

Within matriarchal cultures on Earth, the black ray played an integral part in the practice of earth magic. With the advent of the reign of patriarchal energy, the black ray went underground and people became afraid of it. The patriarchal invaders, in their efforts to dissuade the goddess-based earth philosophies, instilled fear through intimidation within the Celtic, Native American, Mayan, and other shamanic-oriented religions.

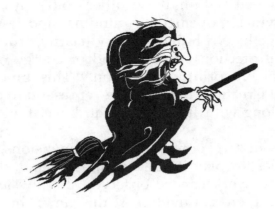

Wiccan practitioners (witches) were portrayed with propagandized lies...dressed in ugly black dresses, casting evil spells and boiling creatures in their cauldrons; all the while scratching the warts on their noses!

In the ancient mystery schools the black ray was called the *unknown*; its qualities were perceived by only a few covert bands of devoted spiritual initiates. In the ancient Druid religions, the high priests and priestesses wore black.

Even today, in many religious organizations, the black robe is a symbol of spiritual attainment and wisdom. Fully trained Catholic priests and nuns wear the black robes.

Perhaps, the black ray's testing and moving qualities have contributed to its bad reputation. People, as a whole, are not enthusiastic about being tested, or moved from, their perspective views of reality. The black ray forces change; it also forces growth. Creation has decreed it to be the force which prevents stagnation. Along the way, the black ray became a kind of test. The movement became a force of determination for people, forcing them to make choices in their lives, be they positive or negative. This, of course, caused fear, resulting from the expected accountability and responsibility for one's actions.

So, how can one use the black ray for healing, especially for healing the planet?

We activate it for purposes of movement, for moving energy blocks (in both our bodies and Mother Earth's body).

All souls have a color ray that they are a part of and vibrate to. Souls who are on the black ray but generally express themselves through one of the other color rays. For example: you may be of the black ray but wish to express healing and love on the green and rose rays. Your aura would be dominated by green and rose, not the thin black line around the outside of your aura's boundary representing the soul energy.

At this time, the black ray is strongly present on Earth to provide stabilization during the planet's shift to the 4th dimension. The black ray helps individual's "clear" their physical body, balance their mental and emotional bodies, and align their spiritual body within the physical body. There is no more time for sitting on the fence. The black ray's intensity is needed to get us moving! The bottom line is, don't be afraid of it; use it to stay *clear* and *balanced*.

The Soul Colors of Manifestation

Color	Attributes/Represents
Red	Deeply physical. Protector/creator of elements: air, fire, water, and earth
Orange	Guardians of physical reality. Guardians of animals, plants, and minerals.
Yellow	Power
Green	Healing and transmutation on the physical level
Rose	Love energy, harmony, and peace
Translucent Blue	Communication and transmutation on the emotional level
Indigo	Scientific data, mental level, the architects
Violet	Spirituality
Silver	Creative energy, feminine aspect
Gold	Active energy, masculine aspect
White	Truth
Clear	Messengers
Black	Testing and grounding

Chart 16-1

The Origin of Creation

Originally, there was the Void, or the Source. It is known in ancient eastern teachings as the Tao, or the blackness. Eventually, from that Void, came a kind of movement. That movement created pure energy, and became known as the four universal laws of Light, Love, Free Will, and Balance. *These universal laws have never changed; they are present throughout all of Creation. They formed what we know as God or the Womb of Creation.*

180

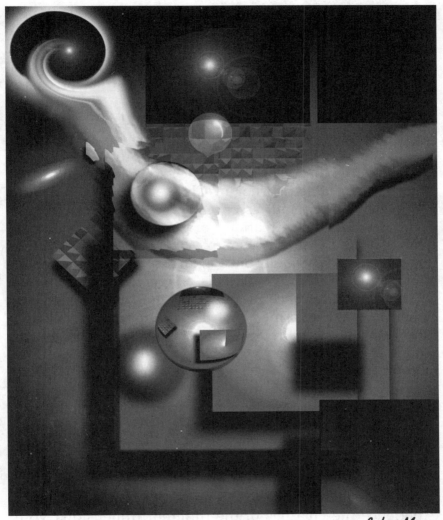

John Mason

There was <u>conscious</u> movement, which created Pure Thought. In other words, the movement wasn't random, but was directed from some higher source. From this came a burst of energy, likened to an explosion, which created the 13 rays and gave color to the Universal Laws. Light became *gold*, Love became *silver*, Free Will was colored *rose*, and Balance was formed by the triad of energy composed of *white, clear,* and *black.*

Again, there was more movement, and what emerged was the creation of the 13 etheric dimensions. They were composed of triads of energies which in turn became the Intent of Creation.

As was explained earlier in Chapter 3, the **Intent** is the blueprint. We, as soul essences, have mirrored our own existences, based on Creation's original set up. The microcosm reflects the macrocosm.

There was movement once again. (My guides have explained that non-movement is a sign of imbalance; the Universe will not accept imbalance.) The non-physical dimensions were formed by triads of energies. This non-physical Universe became the **Data/Expression** of the Source energy. In other words, it carried out the blueprint in terms of certain data, and expression of that data, for the purposes of growth and learning.

Finally, to form the **Physical Manifestation** of the universes, planets, and lifeforms, the 13 seeds of Creation were constructed. Spiritual Intent culminated in the manifestation of physical bodies, both of planets and living beings.

It is possible to tap into all levels of Creation. You can experience the energies of the different dimensions yourself and transfer them to others. The latter part of this chapter gives you the ray combinations that allow you to connect with the blueprints of either the etheric, non-physical, or the physical dimensions as they were being created. It will take practice to become fully acquainted

Waves of Creation

(Original Blueprint)

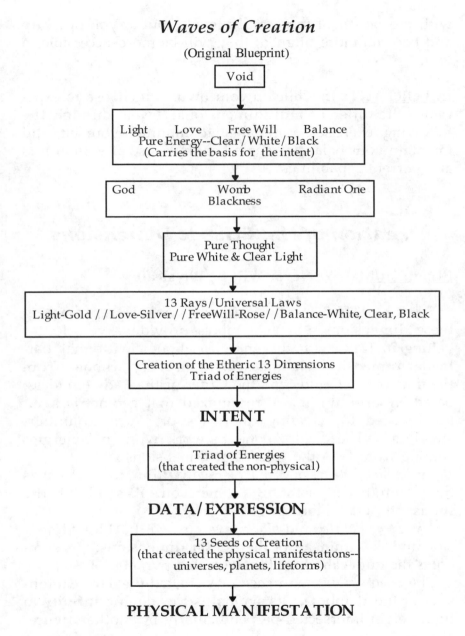

Void

Light   Love   Free Will   Balance
Pure Energy--Clear / White / Black
(Carries the basis for the intent)

God   Womb   Radiant One
Blackness

Pure Thought
Pure White & Clear Light

13 Rays / Universal Laws
Light-Gold / / Love-Silver / / FreeWill-Rose / / Balance-White, Clear, Black

Creation of the Etheric 13 Dimensions
Triad of Energies

INTENT

Triad of Energies
(that created the non-physical)

DATA / EXPRESSION

13 Seeds of Creation
(that created the physical manifestations--
universes, planets, lifeforms)

PHYSICAL MANIFESTATION

Chart 16-2

with the power of these multi-levels, but as you open up and become more aligned, they will be more accessible to you.

IMPORTANT: If, while on your own, you choose to experience the different multidimensional levels through the following exercises, remember to monitor yourself and maintain your balance; keep a healthy sense of your limits and current capabilities.

Creation of the Etheric Dimensions

Blueprint/Matrix (Never Will Be Physical)

See Chart 16-3 for the various symbols representing these dimensions. Such symbols provide a vehicle for getting in tune with the energies aligned with that particular dimension. In the ancient mystery schools, from the time of the Druids and the Order of the Lady (goddess-based philosophy), it was recognized that geometric symbols existed for creating doorways or "keys to understanding". These allow one to work with the energies coming from the other places or dimensions..

The *black, clear,* and *white* rays (within the center) is the womb (black) or the 13th dimension. Its symbol is the **thousand petaled lotus**.

The *clear, white,* and *black* rays created the 12th dimension and is within all of the denser dimensions. Its symbol is the **dodecahedron** (twelve-sided pyramid).

The *clear, violet,* and *rose* rays created the 11th dimension of the Rainbow. Its symbol is the **double infinity** (a figure-eight intersected perpendicularly by another figure-eight).

184

The *white, indigo,* and *yellow* rays created the 10th dimension where the various spiritual orders were formed. Its symbol is the **caduceus**.

The *gold, translucent blue,* and *orange* rays created the 9th dimension where the triad of energies emerged. Its symbol is the **circle**, with the **triangle** inside, and the **square** inside the triangle.

The *silver, green,* and *red* rays created the 8th dimension, where the seeds of creation formed. Its symbol is the **octahedron** (an eight-sided pyramid).

The *black, silver,* and *gold* rays created the 7th dimension, where the beginning movement of the physical began to form. Its symbol is the **spiral**.

The *gold, white,* and *clear* rays created the 6th dimension. Its symbol is the **diamond**.

The *violet, silver,* and *gold* rays created the 5th dimension. Its symbol is the **circle**.

The *translucent blue, indigo,* and *violet* rays created the 4th dimension. Its symbol is the **five-pointed star**.

The *green, rose,* and *translucent blue* rays created the 3rd dimension. Its symbol is the **triangle**.

The *orange, yellow,* and *green* rays created the 2nd dimension. Its symbol is the **medicine wheel** (a cross inside a circle).

The *red, orange,* and *yellow* rays created the 1st dimension. Its symbol is the **cross**.

Symbols & Rays Blueprint

Dimension	Symbol	Ray Colors
1st	Cross 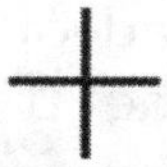 	Red, Orange, Yellow
2nd	Medicine Wheel 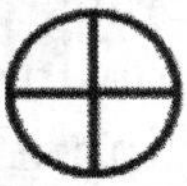 	Orange, Yellow, Green
3rd	Triangle 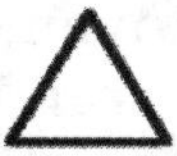 	Green, Rose, Translucent Blue
4th	5 Point Star 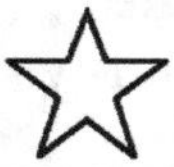 	Translucent Blue, Indigo, Violet
5th	Circle 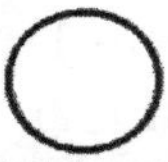 	Violet, Silver, Gold
6th	Diamond 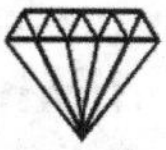 	Gold, White, Clear
7th	Spiral 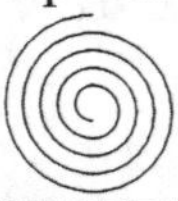 	Black, Silver, Gold

Chart 16-3

Dimension	Symbol	Ray Colors
8th	Octahedron (8 sided crystal) 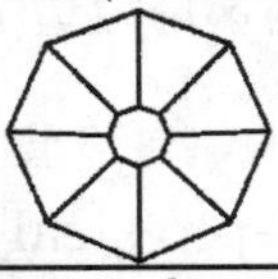	Silver, Green, Red
9th	A square inside a triangle inside a circle 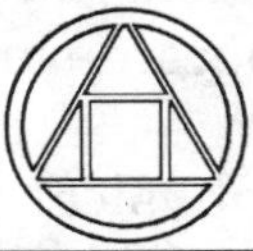	Gold, Translucent Blue, Orange
10th	Cadeusus 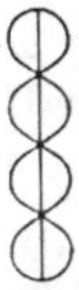	White Indigo, Yellow
11th	Double Infinity 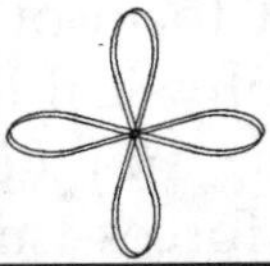	Clear, Violet, Rose
12th	Dodecahedron (12 sided crystal) 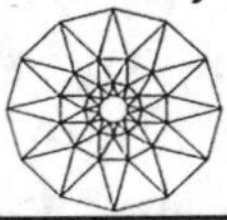	Clear, White, Black
13th	Thousand Petaled Lotus 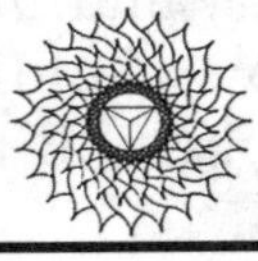	Black (womb), Clear, White (center)

Chart 16-3

Triads of Energies

Triad Combinations of Energies Which Created the Non-Physical:

The **black ray** (at the non-physical level) was created by a combination of *white*, *clear*, and *black* energies. These energies represent the universal laws of Light, Love, Free Will, and Balance. They became the blueprint that embraces all of Creation.

The **clear ray** (at the non-physical level) was created by a combination of *gold*, *clear*, and *black*. These energies represent the universal law of Light, active energy of the Source, the highest form of Light, and the will of Creation.

The **white ray** (at the non-physical level) was created by a combination of *silver*, *clear*, and *black*. These energies represent the universal law of Love, pure spiritual Love from the Source, the highest form of Love.

The **gold ray** (at the non-physical level) was created by a combination of *silver*, *gold*, and *black*. These energies represent the androgynous forces (male and female), and movement.

The **silver ray** (at the non-physical level) was created by a combination of *silver*, *green*, and *violet*. These energies represent the feminine force, alignment, and spirituality.

The **violet ray** (at the non-physical level) was created by a combination of *rose*, *white*, and *violet*. These energies represent unconditional Love (or the emotional expression of the blueprint at the physical level), protection, and spirituality.

The **indigo ray** (at the non-physical level) was created by a combination of *translucent blue*, *indigo*, and *black*. These energies represent communication, logic, active psychic abilities, balance between logic and intuition, and movement.

The **translucent blue ray** (at the non-physical level) was created by a combination of *translucent blue, white,* and *clear.* These energies represent communication, protection, and truth.

The **rose ray** (at the non-physical level) was created by a combination of *rose, clear,* and *yellow.* These energies represent unconditional Love, truth, and power at the physical level.

The **green ray** (at the non-physical level) was created by a combination of *green out of the white ray, green out of the clear ray,* and *green.* These energies represent complete healing at the physical level of all bodies (physical, emotional, mental, and spiritual).

The **yellow ray** (at the non-physical level) was created by a combination of *green, gold,* and *orange.* These energies represent physical healing (at the cellular body), active masculine energies, and creativity at the physical levels.

The **orange ray** (at the non-physical level) was created by a combination of *green, orange,* and *red.* These energies represent the devic energies, healing at the physical level (physical body), creativity at the physical levels, and the heaviest (or densest) physical energies.

The **red ray** (at the non-physical level) was created by a combination of *red out of the black ray, red out of the white ray,* and *red.* These energies represent the heaviest (densest) physical energies.

The Seeds of Creation

My spiritual guides have given me information regarding the way Creation was formed at every dimensional level. The following recreates the formation of the Universe at the physical level.

Physical Level--The Role and Participation in Creation, the Gifts, the Purpose

Imagine the Creative Womb akin to a primordial Ocean. This Ocean gathered momentum, movement, and energy through the contrasting forces of Light, Love, Free Will, and Balance (the four basic elemental energies which have been duplicated throughout Creation). At the time of Creation of the physical universe, these forces created a spiraling energy in this Ocean called the Womb; this caused movement to spring outward from It. That movement was defined as "waves", just as the ocean presently moves waves onto the land.

During the **first wave** to create the physical level, the three rays of color were *silver, gold,* and *clear.* The *silver* ray signified multiple preservation and female polarity. The *gold* signified active spiritual knowledge and male polarity. The *clear* ray was the "messenger" between the rays and the Womb of Creation. Together, they created the *non-physical, spiritual* level.

During the **second wave** to create the physical level, the three rays of color were *white, violet,* and *indigo.* The *white* brought forth the search for truth. It created the auras of planets and planetary systems. The *white* ray was the preserver of Truth at all levels. The *violet* brought forth the knowledge of the spiritual lessons, passive spiritual knowledge. The indigo was the architect of the Plan; it brought forth scientific knowledge and abilities. All together, they created the second wave of the *non-physical, spiritual* level.

During the **third wave** to create the physical level, the three rays of color were *translucent blue, rose,* and *green.* The *translucent blue* brought forth the emotional aspect of the systems; it was the transformer of the spiritual to the physical, the collector of knowledge. The *rose* brought

190

forth harmony, balance, different colors, textures, and sounds. It also preserved healing and unconditional Love. The *green* became record keeper of earth history, and aided healing in plant and animal life. *Green* also brought movement into the physical levels. All together, they created the ***non-physical, emotional*** level.

During the **fourth wave** to create the physical level, the three rays of color were *yellow, orange,* and *red*. The *yellow* was the impetus that solidified everything; it was the active masculine energy at the physical level. The *orange* was the guardian of plants, minerals, and animals. It became the emotional and the feminine energies at the physical level. The *red* brought forth the movement; it combined male and female energies. All together, they created the ***physical at the physical*** level.

During the **fifth wave** to create the physical level, one ray was used. It was commonly known as the <u>unknown</u> or the *black* ray. Its purpose was to provide protection on the physical level, grounding, and testing. Its function became movement. It appeared on all of the dimensional levels...from ***the etheric, or spiritual level, to the densest physical level***, our own.

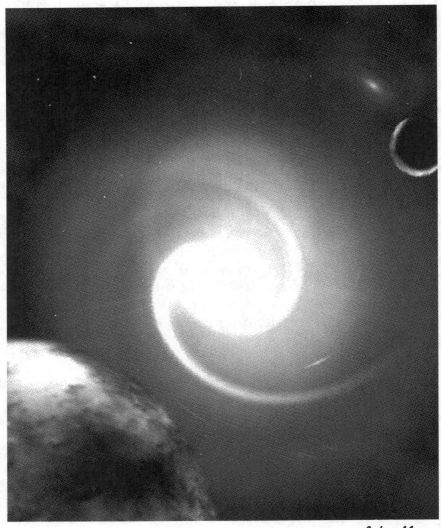

John Mason

Chapter 17

Connecting to the Source

═══════════════════════════════════

Come Dance the Rainbow on Wings of Love

There are wings of Light that flow ever forward;
They bring the dance.

The dance of two shall join to unite the color,
And the color shall move.

Movement will bring two as one,
The one will bring the Rainbow

Come dance the Rainbow on wings of Love
As one.

--- *Adassan*
1990

13 Rays Exercise

The legends of ancient cultures speak of a distant future (with some indication that 1993 was a pivotal year for an awakening) when individuals, known as the *Rainbow Warriors*, would come from different races, cultures, and economic backgrounds. They will have unique communication abilities; they will form *rainbow tribes* as they become beacons of Light. The Rainbow Warriors will facilitate healing for planet Earth, allowing it to become more healthy and peaceful.

Purpose: This rainbow energy exists throughout Creation. The following specific technique will introduce you to the totality of different colors available from the Source.

- Bring the *black* ray into your body through your crown chakra. Have it flow down into your hands.
- From your hands, make a braid* of the 13 rays, one-at-at-time, starting with the *red* ray. Then, braid in the *orange, yellow, green, rose, translucent blue, indigo, purple, white, silver, gold,* and *clear*. These will be combined with the *black* ray.
- With a partner, place your hand at his/her base chakra (at the base of the spine); place your other hand at the medulla oblongata (back of the neck at the base of the skull).
- Channel the braided 13 rays of energy into these receptive points.
- As with all energy techniques, let the extra energy dissipate; when you are finished clear and ground your-

---

* A *braid* is defined as "three or more links of energy or rays woven together to a particular point."

self. Make sure your partner also grounds himself or herself.

Alignment Technique

Purpose: To connect you directly to your spirit, or Higher Self.

- Sit cross-legged on the floor. Press your palms against the floor. (Fig. 17.1a)
- Draw *silver* energy from the center of the earth. Move it upward. Place your right hand in front of your heart chakra, with your palm facing the left side of your body as the silver is being *run*. (Fig. 17.1b)

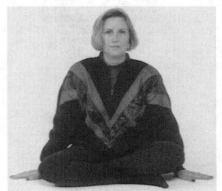 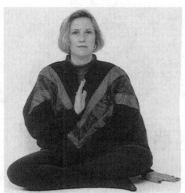

Fig. 17.1a   Fig. 17.1b

- Continue to run the *silver* as you bring *gold* down from the heavens. As you channel the gold, bring your left hand from the floor, raise it above the head, then bring it down to the heart chakra in one fluid motion. Your left palm should be facing the other palm. (Fig. 17.1c)
- Allow the gold and silver to continue to flow. Now stretch both arms overhead, close together, as you bring forth the clear ray. (Fig. 17.1d)

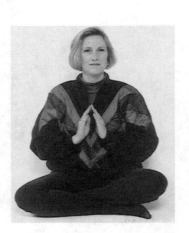

Fig. 17.1c

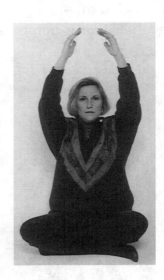

Fig. 17.1d

- Add *white*, as you keep your arms overhead while holding your arms about 18 inches apart. (Fig. 17.1e)
- Next, add *black* as you move your arms about a yard apart. (Fig. 17.1f)
- Then bring that combined energy fully down into your body to align it. Both hands are brought down at the same time from the last position to the heart chakra with your palms placed together. (Fig. 17.1g)

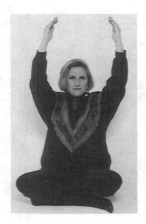

Fig. 17.1e

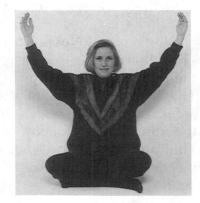

Fig. 17.1f

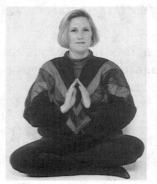

Fig. 17.1g

Clearing Blocks Exercise

Purpose: To facilitate a link from the physical, emotional, and mental bodies to the spiritual body.

When sending a healing ray to someone (such as emerald green):
1) Add the *white ray* for protection.
2) Add the *clear ray*. (This will help you determine what the imbalance is.)
3) Add the *black ray* to create movement.

Notes To Remember
- The **etheric** level never comes into the physical. It is the *Intent*, or the blueprint ... the spiritual body.
- The intent registers in the mental/emotional (which are the *data/expression* levels), otherwise known as the **non-physical** planes of existence.
- The **physical** is the *manifestation* of the Intent...the physical body.

Discovering Your Intent

Purpose: To reach a meditative/visualization state. To gain information regarding your soul ray, as well as the ray you are currently expressing.

Procedure:
- Visualize each chakra as it changes from its normal color to *violet*. (Start at the base chakra and work upward to the crown.)
- Next, spiritually create a vortex of violet energy around your head area and move into the center of it.

198

When you're in the center of the vortex, you are in the causal realm.

- Ask your Higher Self, or your guides, to reveal the color of your soul ray.
- Now, visualize your aura colors; and ask for the color of the ray you are currently expressing, in the here and now of the present dimension.
- With color, define your intent for being here. Which color ray represents your:
    - a) Spiritual Intent
    - b) Mental Data/Emotional Expression
    - c) Physical Manifestation

Braiding the 13 Rays to the Source

Purpose: To connect your essence in a *conscious* way (we are never apart from It) to the Eternal Being.

Procedure: (Prior to doing this exercise, be sure that you have first grounded.)

- Bring in the *silver* ray through your feet; this will connect you to Mother Earth.
- From the Source, bring the *gold* ray through your crown chakra; this will connect you to what we call God.
- Now, braid your **base chakra** to the Source by sending It a cord of *red*, *gold*, and *silver* (originating from your base chakra).
- Braid your **spleen chakra** to the Source by sending It a cord of *orange*, *gold*, and *silver* (originating from your spleen chakra).

- Braid your **solar plexus chakra** to the Source by sending It a cord of *yellow, gold,* and *silver* (originating from your solar plexus chakra).
- Braid your **heart chakra** to the Source by sending It a cord of *green, rose, gold,* and *silver* (originating from your heart chakra).
- Braid your **throat chakra** to the Source by sending It a cord of *translucent blue, gold* and *silver* (originating from your throat chakra).
- Braid your **third eye** to the Source by sending a cord of *indigo, gold,* and *silver* (originating from your third eye chakra).
- Braid your **crown chakra** to the Source by sending It a cord of *violet, gold,* and *silver* (originating from your crown chakra).
- Connect to the Source by sending It a cord of *silver* from your **silver chakra** below the feet.
- Connect to the Source by sending It a cord of *gold* from your **gold chakra** above the head.
- Connect to the Source by sending It a cord of *white* from your **white chakra** in the palm of your dominant hand.
- Connect to the Source by sending It a cord of *clear* energy from your **clear chakra** in the palm of your non-dominant hand.
- Connect to the Source by sending It a cord of *black* from the **black chakra** below the feet (located under the silver chakra).
- Solidly ground following this exercise!

Aspects of the Source

Within the Source, there is no time or space. It exists in the Eternal Now. It does, however, recognize aspects or traits, and we can tap into each one of them. Generally, we choose to express a particular trait in our physical or non-physical lifetimes. These aspects of ourselves change with each lifetime, and are linked to the 13 rays of color.

To determine which aspects you have decided to express throughout your lifetimes, relax into a deep state of meditation. You may use any of the visualization or meditation techniques I have already mentioned. Ask your Higher Self, your guides, or even the Source, which aspect of the Source your soul has chosen to express.

	Aspect	Ray
1	Birth	Red
2	Understanding	Orange
3	Homogeny	Yellow
4	Knowledge	Green
5	Emotion	Rose
6	Clarity	Translucent Blue
7	Wisdom	Indigo
8	Service	Purple
9	Completion	Silver
10	Mastery	Gold
11	Unfoldment	White
12	Creation	Clear
13	One	Black

Solar Plexus Tying

The purpose of this technique is to give you a "first aid" energy tool, one which we have successfully used in serious cases where strong measures were required. (This approach should be used <u>only</u> in emergencies, for no more than 48 hours. While it is in process, stay alert to your own body for this technique can be very draining.)

Practice this technique with a partner when there is no emergency to accustom yourself to the process before it is needed. While you work together, stay aware as you tune into the sensations of connecting in this manner. Keep the connection for **a few minutes only**. Unless one of you is ill, or very imbalanced, there should be no detrimental effects with this type of short-term connection.

The technique is as follows:

- Sit facing opposite one another. Choose who will go first.
- The transmitter brings from his/her solar plexus a *gold, silver,* and *yellow* cord.

  The transmitter mentally "braids" these rays into the **solar plexus** of the partner. This process facilitates a healing connection for anyone who is ill.
- Share your intuitive observations of being connected with one another.
- Dissipate the energy connection.
- Exchange roles.
- When complete, make sure <u>all</u> the energy is dissipated. Clear and ground.

Tying Into all of the Chakras

With a partner (who is also studying this book) you may tie into all of each other's chakras. As I stated in the Solar Plexus Tying exercise, this is not a technique to be used carelessly.

Rather than for healing purposes, I would like you to do this exercise specifically for the bonding experience. **It is to be done for no longer than 15 minutes at a time.**

Important: Not to be done if either is physically ill, emotionally, mentally, or spiritually out of balance.

- Make sure you have grounded, protected, and balanced your chakras prior to starting.
- Sit in a chair facing your partner. Greet him/her in "the Love and Light of Creation."
- Braid the *gold, silver* and *red* rays together at your base chakra and send this cord out to your partner's **base chakra**.
- Braid the *gold, silver,* and *orange* rays together at your spleen chakra and send this cord out to your partner's **spleen chakra**.
- Braid the *gold, silver,* and *yellow* rays together at your solar plexus chakra and send this cord out to your partner's **solar plexus**.
- Braid the *gold, silver,* and *green* rays together at your heart chakra and send this cord out to your partner's **heart chakra**.
- Braid the *gold, silver,* and *translucent blue* rays together at your throat chakra and send this cord out to your partner's **throat chakra**.
- Braid the *gold, silver,* and *indigo* rays together at your third eye chakra and send this cord out to your partner's **third eye**.

- Braid the *gold, silver,* and *purple* rays together at your crown chakra and send this cord out to your partner's **crown**.
- Note the feelings or sensations within each chakra.
- Let the braids dissipate. <u>Clear,</u> ground, and balance.

Note: If the braids are not unlinked, you invite severe depletion of your life force energy. This happened to me. While facilitating a new "walk-in"[*] I left my chakra braids linked-in for approximately nine days. It depleted me to such an extent that I ended up in the hospital emergency room two times with a severe case of hives. My face was almost unrecognizable due to extreme swelling. My immune system suffered to such a degree that it took approximately 1 1/2 years for it to return to normal.

---

[*] A soul exchange (See Glossary for explanation.)

Chapter 18

Strengths and Weaknesses of a Healer

===

"The most terrifying thing is to accept oneself completely."

--Carl Jung

Physical, Emotional, and Mental Assets and Liabilities

This is a self-evaluation of who you are at this moment of your life. Please honestly evaluate your strengths and weaknesses in each category:

Physical

Strengths   _____

_____

_____

Weaknesses   _____

_____

_____

Emotional

Strengths   _____

_____

_____

Weaknesses   _____

_____

_____

Mental

Strengths

_____

_____

_____

Weaknesses

_____

_____

_____

As a Healer

Strengths

_____

_____

_____

Weaknesses

_____

_____

_____

When you have completed the previous pages, you may study this example for insight.

Examples of Strengths and Weaknesses:

Physical

Strengths — Good physical body, regular exercise, vitamins and/or herbs daily, good quality food intake, cleansing diet, frequent Epsom salt/vinegar baths, sufficient water intake.

Weaknesses — Regular junk food intake, including excessive sugar, or food bingeing, immune system weakness and/or other physical disease.

Emotional

Strengths — Balanced, stable, grounded, empathic, have resolved major life issues, is "clearing" well, open heart chakra, willingness to open locked emotional doors, willingness to allow energies to flow through you.

Weaknesses   Emotional instability, attachments to certain outcomes, "hidden agendas", mirroring, "stuffing" emotions, oversensitivity, irrational emoting (high drama), insecurities.

Mental

Strengths   Will power, intuition, clarity of thought, open-mindedness, logic, analytical, balanced perspective, avid reader, writer, highly visual.

Weaknesses   Mental stress, doubts, fears, dyslexia and other learning disabilities, memory problems, close-minded, inability to concentrate or focus.

As a Healer

Strengths   Healing experience, good channel, empathic, masculine and feminine balance, knowledge of anatomy, responsible healer, "clean" energy channel, knows how to build a support group of healers, knowledge of multiple modalities, can set up a referral network.

Weaknesses — Over-empathetic, sympathetic versus empathetic, not enough relaxation, doubt of personal abilities, blind spots such as not knowing one's self, the four "deadly sins" -- egotism, greed, fear, adultery (not the sexual meaning but to go against your conscience by altering yourself or another person), attached to outcomes.

Chapter 19

Alchemy and the Holographic Universe

═══════════════════════════

Alchemist's Log

Two ounces of light
A hair from the dog
A pound of lead
An infusion of fog
Six words in French
Two words in Greek
And lo we have gold.

-St. Germain

A Holographic Vs. Linear Perspective

There is a revolution in spiritual consciousness taking place in our world right now, a revolution that has been building for several decades. It represents a quantum shift in our perceptions, our awareness of the intimate link to our souls or inner selves, to our brothers and sisters, and to all living beings. This revolution in consciousness demands changes in our archaic "tunnel-vision" views of reality, it requires that we embrace the larger picture, a *Holographic Perspective*.

This is a new cutting-edge theory of philosophy presented by Stanislov Grof, who calls it the "holographic mind" or the "holographic universe." Holography is a photographic process that uses laser-coherent light of the same wavelength to produce three-dimensional images in space. As a result of this technology, a complete three-dimensional image can be "unfolded" from any fraction of the hologram. It can be cut into many pieces and each part will still be capable of reproducing an image of the whole.

The Holographic Perspective is a **complete** multidimensional frame of reference as opposed to a linear or flat perspective of reality. Altering a single component of the holograph simultaneously alters every other component within it. As we evolve, we change the holograph by our shifts in consciousness, creating a distinctly different "picture". This impacts all of Creation. From this perspective, the holograph is in constant flux, reflecting the balance or imbalance within the universe.

Within the Holographic Universe, we are all One. Because of this, it is important that we be in a constant state of integrity, not only with ourselves, but with one another. Remember, what we are, do, and think impacts

212

everyone. We must even take responsibility for all of the emotions we feel.

The key to evolution is your willingness to become self-empowered, to see yourself as the *cause* rather than the *effect*. The degree to which you feel "in charge" of your life affects your ability to create your own reality. Important in all this is your willingness to assume responsibility for your own life, to acknowledge that you are presented with constant choices, and have the final say in what happens. Seeing yourself as a victim is a "cop-out", as is blaming others for the outcome.

As we ground, clear, balance, and protect our energies, we allow a process to occur whereby we can begin to infuse our bodies (the physical, mental, and emotional) with spiritual energy, thus clearing ourselves of unwanted negative patterns.

Spiritual energy is comprised of two aspects: the masculine principle, and the feminine standard. On a spiritual level, the masculine energies express predominantly through the *physical* and *mental* bodies; the feminine energies express predominantly through the *spiritual* and *emotional* bodies.

The masculine energies tend to be **self-serving**, while the feminine energies tend to be more **selfless** in nature. Also, expressed through the masculine and feminine principles is the duality of giving and receiving. Inherent to the feminine standard is the desire to heal, and the counterpart in the masculine dynamic is the action-orientation that creates movement.

Using the breath as a way to connect spiritually is not as valid as we have been led to believe. In the yogic tradition, some feel that the "breath of life," or *prana*, comes into the body through the lungs. This is a misconception, but it works for those who practice this procedure, due to the strength of the belief system that surrounds this practice.

In reality, spiritual energies move into the physical body through the chakra system.

Contained within the chakra system is the genetic coding that connects us to our evolutionary past, our dynamic present, and our probable future. Using various techniques, it is possible to activate that genetic coding, setting up a dynamic for the unfolding of <u>all</u> that we are.

While practicing these techniques, you as the practitioner, will strengthen your ties to the various kingdoms (animal, vegetable, and mineral), planets, and universes.

These exercises will allow you to quickly access who you truly are. Simultaneously, with this you will increase your vibrational rate, your ability to heal, and your power to manifest what you really want.

In short, the primary intention is to assist you in moving from a linear self of limited understanding to a holographic or multidimensional sense of who you are.

Along with this, as you move the spiritual energies through the chakra system and into the physical, mental, and emotional bodies, you can begin to consciously activate your gifts, talents, and extrasensory abilities.

I have come to realize that the glands and organs of the physical body have metaphysical properties or functions. Very few of us have an awareness of these metaphysical functions.

In Chapter 24, I shall define which glands or organs are connected with a particular psychic gift, (such as the appendix being the seat of telepathy), and how to activate or sharpen that specific ability. As Ken Carey states in his book, <u>Starseed, The Third Millennium</u>, published in 1991: "These glands [in the endocrine system] bridge spirit and matter. They are the biologic receptors that translate the higher-frequency information picked up by the etheric disks (the chakras of yogic tradition) into language the nervous system can recognize. They are designated to audit ultrafine frequencies, bringing both sensory and what some would call extrasensory impressions into your awareness."

The building blocks of our work are the masculine and feminine energies; that is, balancing and merging them within the chakra system, and the physical, mental, and emotional bodies.

When we incorporate all of the other aspects of who we are (mineral, plant, animal, angelic), we begin to move beyond concepts of space and time and we are capable of fully embracing our many dimensional nature. When we bring the planetary and star energy into our chakra system we are fully able to encompass our God-like nature. All of our aspects and multidimensional selves merge into one totality, although we still have an awareness--in space and time--of this particular embodiment. With this level of awareness, which is 14th dimensional in nature, we can simultaneously embrace a particular experience or incident in our lives; we can overlay it with who we are dimensionally.

As we equally envelop spirit, energy, and matter on a spiritual level, truth versus illusion on a mental level, love versus fear on an emotional level, unlimitedness versus limitedness on a physical level, we begin to access states of Christ and cosmic consciousness.

In summary, the linear experience of our reality limits our understanding of ourselves as interdimensional spiritual beings. *The sum of who we are includes numerous multiple selves on many different dimensions.* Our 3rd plane existence has encased what the shamans call *monochronic* time (a rigid concept of past, present, and future) as all there is. The holographic experience views our existence as multidimensional, multi-aspected, one that moves within a fluid framework of *polychronic* time (a non-linear, quantum, "Eternal Now" with multiple realities).

The Holographic Universe Process

Purpose: To shift from the *linear* you into the *quantum* you. A penetrating, potentially quick way of accessing and clearing deeply ingrained patterns, phobias, and traumas.

This technique is best done in a group of no less than six people. Four people will play the "bodies," one will facilitate, and one will be processor.

Procedure:
- Before starting, everyone present should ground, protect, and balance their chakras.
- You, the processor, decide what you wish to "clear" or work on. If nothing obvious comes up, you can just go ahead with the technique and see what surfaces.
- Now, determine which person present you would like to play the part of your *physical* body, who you would like to have as your *emotional* body, who you would like to represent your *mental* body, and who you want to play your *spiritual* body. These participants will intuitively reflect the energy of the body they are chosen to play. The facilitator should be experienced in the Holographic Universe technique and with potentially traumatic situations. He or she will monitor all of the participants. It is imperative that the facilitator maintain a cool head and an experienced, soothing, healing presence.

Realize that even if you are not the designated *processor*, **you may also do personal processing. This technique usually impacts** <u>all</u> **of the participants while bringing up their own issues or traumas. Remember, in the holographic space there are no coincidences. Every aspect is important and contributes to the whole.**

- As processor, determine where you will begin. It's up to you to choose. You may start from the physical body position (see Chart 19-1 for direction), the emotional body position, the mental body position, or the spiritual (soul) position. Go to that position. You may stand or sit, whichever is more comfortable.

- Ask that particular *body* (designated person) for its impressions of the particular issue. If there is no apparent issue on the table, just allow the viewpoints to come forth. The person playing the body should always state his/her opinions in the third person. In other words, when expressing a feeling or perception, one should say, for example, "<u>W</u> e feel a sadness in the heart area," rather than, "<u>I</u> feel a sadness in the heart area."

- When, for the moment, that particular body is finished, intuitively go to the next body and allow for the same process to occur.

- Eventually, all four bodies will have a chance to speak. Some of the bodies may have more input than the others; it depends on the issue at hand.

NOTE: In actuality, this technique is less formal than its description. In practice, it becomes a sharing, a give-and-take, a conversation between the processor and the various bodies. More often than not, you will also find that this will include a certain degree of emotionalism or mental intensity. This holographic process will definitely trigger issues needing to be cleared.

Moving from the Linear You to the Quantum You

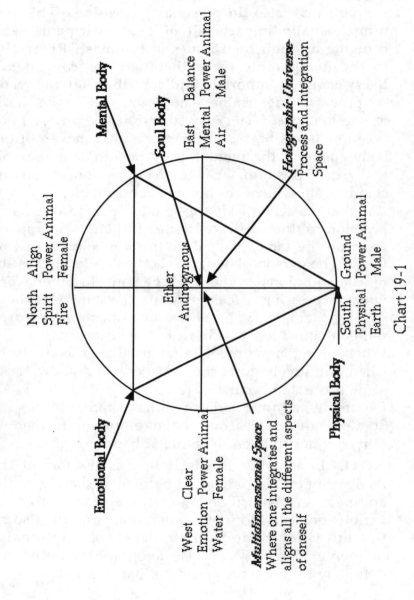

Mental Body

Soul Body

East Balance
Mental Power Animal
Air Male

Holographic Universe
Process and Integration
Space

North Align
Spirit Power Animal
Fire Female

Ether
Androgynous

South Ground
Physical Power Animal
Earth Male

Physical Body

Emotional Body

West Clear
Emotion Power Animal
Water Female

Multidimensional Space
Where one integrates and
aligns all the different aspects
of oneself

Chart 19-1

218

- When all four bodies feel complete in their communication, the processor goes to the center of the circle. The people playing the bodies will surround the processor in a symbolic merging of the physical, emotional, mental, and spiritual bodies.
- Finish the exercise with a supportive group hug.
- Be sure that all participants ground and re-balance their chakras.

What is Alchemy?

Webster's Dictionary defines **alchemy** as "the chemistry of the middle ages, the chief aim of which was to change the baser elements into gold." This is only one aspect of alchemy. The clear-visioned alchemists of the middle ages and Renaissance time periods, such as St. Germain and Paracelsus, knew alchemy's more interesting application as a tool for self-transformation.

The art and science of alchemy is a purification process. The alchemist knows how to condense the strength found in the plant kingdom, understands how to improve the value of minerals from this and other planets (including turning lead into gold). The alchemist develops the value of stones from this and other planes, and comprehends how to make fine jewels from baser elements and flawed crystals. Except for healing purposes, the alchemist rarely intrudes on the animal kingdom. He/She understands how to harness the power of the elements for transformation and protection, while simultaneously increasing the purity and value of their essences.

Alchemy can be applied to the physical workings of turning lead into gold as well as the psychological process of transformation. Purification is the emphasis, a focus that attains refinement of the physical and psychic. Both processes pursue **pure essence**.

The alchemist concentrates on the relationship between the elements: earth, air, fire, water, and ether. This concentration of energy is focused on the relationship between body, emotions, mind, and the perfection of the soul. There are three main stages of alchemical work: *separation, purification,* and *recombination.*

The process of **distillation** is separation. The physical alchemical process breaks down a plant and heats its matter, releasing its essence. In the psychological alchemical process, distillation requires the breaking down and destruction of useless attitudes or negative patterns; these ideas alienate us from the God-Self.

Distillation leaves us with a more purified image of ourselves. We step further into the metaphysical, allowing the distillation process to take place within our own *four bodies*--physical, emotional, mental, and spiritual. We, in effect, become our own laboratories. These four bodies act as our "tools" along with the elements, the planets, the universes, and the multiple dimensions. As part of this process, crystals, chakras, medicine shields, chalices, and swords take on a special, spiritual symbolism; they become providers of power, healing, wealth, peace, and serenity.

Each time the distillation process takes place you take a step forward. You learn to identify with your soul essence rather than your personality. You stretch the outer boundaries and perceive new, expansive levels of consciousness. At the same time, in the physical alchemical laboratory, matter is purged of its denseness. This is the **solutio** or liquid process.

Sublimatio, or purification, is the interaction of air or gas. This is an uplifting process that transforms a condensed substance into one that's less dense. This can happen within the alchemical lab or within the individual psyche. The soul is temporarily removed from the earth plane; it soars unencumbered in meditation, as it catches glimpses of immortality, walks through walls, and examines the underpinning of teleportation through the physical realm. Sublimation (sublimato), an extraction process, also leads to out-of-body soul travel and other cosmic states of awareness.

Coagulatio, or recombination, is the condensation of purified, compressed substances while working in the alchemical lab. When pursuing a transformation of the psyche, the same result occurs. A new, purely refined essence results from both processes.

For the individual, there may be a choice to be made, whether or not to continue dwelling upon the 3rd plane of Earth. As one passes through this process an opportunity is offered for a reunion with Source. This self-realization state of consciousness may be immediately known, or many more rounds of distillation may be required. Coagulatio is the reconnection with a more harmonious, yet grounded lifestyle. In this spiritual state we are released from a limited personal view, and connected for a time with our guides and a more holistic viewpoint. For example, on a physical alchemical level, this state is one in which a concentrated, highly refined product (such as the essential oil rose otto) is produced. This product is very valuable, highly concentrated, and extremely pure in nature.

Natural forces, such as gravity, antigravity, some matter, and antimatter fall beyond human visual perception; they are also difficult concepts for the average psyche to understand. When we incorporate and activate these forces we become the true alchemists that we were intended to be. Likewise, we are better able to understand our observer/participant nature, more cognizant of the mysteries of life, and our own greatness.

In addition, (in our own mind) we seem to be relatively insignificant in the grand scheme of it all, like a grain of sand on a beach. Never underestimate the unfolding empowerment that can evolve from that perspective, should we choose to fully encompass that infinitesimal aspect of ourselves. We are the mystery of our own creation while we simultaneously create our own reality. *We are the macrocosm and we are the microcosm.*

The Alchemical Rays of Creation

In terms of the macrocosm of Creation, I have recently had the privilege to obtain data on the *alchemical* rays.

This information differs somewhat from the blended rays of Chapter 14, wherein the energies of two rays are blended together to create a *composite energy*, or mixture. Blended rays can be distilled (separated) from the over-all composite, even in their pure state.

Alchemical rays have blended together to form a compound which modifies the structure, making it nearly impossible to separate the original, individual rays from the primary combination.

The original 13 rays came singly out of Creation. Over "time," as dimensions and universes have been birthed and become evolved, so some of the rays have begun to blend together. Through the process of evolution they have become rays in their own right. Although the 13 rays of Creation have often banded with each other in twos, or in triads of combined power, to form dimensions of varying vibration, the alchemical rays were created by the original 13 to empower the process of Creation.

I recently received channeled information regarding the original 13 dimensions. Because of the universal desire to evolve, there are now 33 dimensions. The 14th through the 23rd planes are considered the *shadow* dimensions. The 24th through the 33rd planes are called the *quantum* dimensions.

The first 11 dimensions are considered energetically positive, the 12th and 13th are neutral, the 14th through 23rd are considered energetically negative, and the 24th through the 33rd are a blend of both negative and positive.

The original 13 rays, in triads of energy, created the first 13 dimensions. The alchemical blended rays created the shadow and the quantum dimensions. Although these alchemical rays seem to belong exclusively to the 14th through 33rd dimensions, they are also used on the first 13 planes.

In summary, the alchemical rays form new symbolic planes, new universes which are an extension of, but are separate from, the original thirteen.

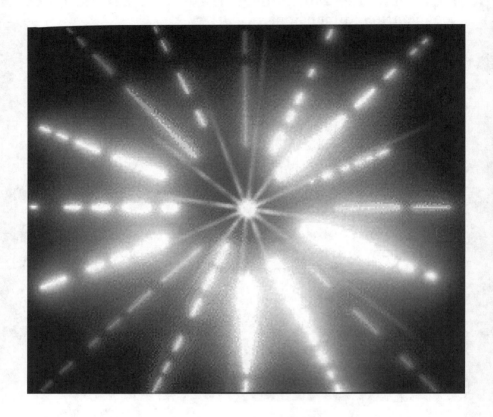

Chapter 20

Advanced Chakra Techniques

"If the doors of perception were cleansed, everything would appear to man as it is, infinite."

---William Blake

A Deeper Look at the Chakras

Now that you have a working understanding of the chakra system, let's delve a little further in comprehending their importance and potential.

Base Chakra

The base chakra's energy is grounded in raw power. When the 1st chakra is "open" you feel abundant, in good health, and connected with your body. Qualities commonly connected with the first chakra are willpower, determination to succeed, leadership, and independence. Traditionally, it has been viewed as a strong masculine energy, linking to the Father principle. However, without the feminine principle working within you at this level, your personality can be bombastic, overbearing, and self-important. Many corporate leaders, past and present, have been "stuck" in this kind of energy.

An imbalance of base chakra energy can create a tendency to see things in terms of "black or white" with an overwhelming desire to acquire material possessions. The overriding feminine quality at the base chakra is vanity. One appreciates superficial beauty (ignoring inner beauty) while being centered on self and focused on acceptance by others.

Spleen Chakra

This chakra is predominantly feminine. When the 2nd chakra is aligned one feels connected to other people, but balances it with time alone. The predominant qualities of the spleen chakra are creativity and confident self-expression. The principle soul quality related to this chakra is intention. Its masculine aspect is one that makes people fall in love. Adaptability and flexibility are also associated with this chakra when the masculine and feminine energies are in balance, implying the ability to take on new challenges. This chakra is related to procreation, bringing forth new life; the counterpoint at this level would be the fear of death. The spleen chakra's negative aspects include killing creativity via fear, anger, jealousy, as well as, the suppression of self-expression.

Solar Plexus Chakra

The primary spiritual expression at this level is free will. Although love-centeredness comes from the heart chakra, the spark comes from the solar plexus. This gives you the strength to sustain through the "thick or thin" of crises. One feminine aspect of the third chakra is the ability to hold the energy; many women do this in the context of the family dynamic. Negative aspects include blind rage and destructive anger. Emotions can be contradictory, raw and animal-like on one hand while serene and poetic on the other. The 3rd chakra is feeling-based, offering usable personal power and emotional control.

Negative aspects of the solar plexus chakra can sometimes be seen in women, many of whom remain immature, "shut down", and relatively undeveloped. On the positive side, blind rage can be used to protect one's country, as demonstrated by Winston Churchill. A mother can also constructively channel the same emotion towards caring for her child, like the mother lion who protects her cubs.

Heart Chakra

The 4th chakra is one of balance and harmony, composed of the highly spiritual qualities of compassion and love. When this chakra is open, and the masculine and feminine are balanced, one feels safe, is able to trust, take risks, love, and feel loved. This chakra's primary feminine quality is courage.

Throat Chakra

When the throat chakra is open, you are able speak your truth with clarity, and express your true feelings with love. The 5th chakra is the center of divine love. The masculine and feminine spiritual energies are merged and balanced here, combining power with knowledge and understanding. At the throat lies the center of wisdom and the power of voice. When the masculine and feminine are balanced here, your speech reflects the perfect balance that is possible. There is a fear of death associated with this center, yet, the overriding polarities expressed are love versus fear, and courage versus cowardice.

Third Eye Chakra

The sixth chakra opens your psychic and intuitive abilities. One can also receive physical and spiritual understanding at the third eye. Mental flexibility acts as a stabilizing force. The third eye is known for its sense of power and acquisition, as a place of knowledge and understanding.

Crown Chakra

The crown chakra is the Spirit center; this definition goes beyond divine wisdom. The crown chakra allows you to connect with the Godhead at the 14th dimension, allowing the Light of the Source to come into your energy field. This chakra is also your connection to your Higher Self, as well as to other dimensions. The crown chakra is a source of imagination and inspiration.

Silver Chakra

Below the feet is the 8th chakra tying you to Mother Earth. It is the feminine balancing energy to the masculine gold ray. It's the transformational energy that you find in nature, a basic kinesthetic knowledge, a doorway to parallel dimensions. The silver chakra amplifies the alchemical nature of the gold ray. At this chakra lies the possibility for one to shapeshift.

Gold Chakra

Above the crown is the 9th chakra. It is the masculine balancing energy for the feminine silver ray. You need the gold chakra to sustain power whenever you move into other dimensions. It amplifies the alchemical nature of the silver ray. The gold ray's power is self-intuitive.

White Chakra

This chakra is located in the palm of the dominant hand; it is the 10th chakra, one that offers a layer of invisible protection. One can liken this protective armor to a selective *Teflon® shield*, one that will deflect evil or negative energy. The white ray is a "power center" for healing. This ray allows you to transform and transmute; it can be effectively utilized after the black ray has already broken through an energy block. In addition, the white ray allows you to move into other dimensions quickly and easily.

Clear Chakra

This is the 11th chakra; it is located in the palm of the non-dominant hand. The essence of the clear chakra is truth and clarity. You could liken it to a mirror where you can clearly see yourself with all of your blemishes and shortcomings. With this chakra point's clear ray one can merge and collapse all of the universes. At this chakra, there is a sense of acuity and mental clarity that can be amped up by a factor of $10 \times 10 \times 10$. This ray's signature is wholeness, completion, and perfection.

Black Chakra

The black chakra is the 12th chakra (or 13th if you count two aspects at the heart chakra). It is located approximately 6" below the feet, surrounding the outer layer of the aura like an envelope. It is the energy of the Tao, from which everything springs, like a fountain of water. The feminine aspect of the black chakra is the movement in, and the masculine aspect is the movement out. This ray is extremely powerful when used for psychic surgery; it allows you to get to the core of a problem quickly and easily. The black ray also embodies the universal androgynous element, or "neutral space." Buddha is an excellent historical example of the black ray energy.

Connecting Your Chakras to the Earth, the Sun, and the Moon

Purpose: To link you consciously to our Earth and the two main celestial bodies essential to its functioning. To expand your awareness, facilitate self-empowerment and a deep alignment with our Creator.

Procedure:
• Turn all 13 chakras 13 times in each direction, first clockwise, then counter-clockwise.
• Tie all of your 13 chakras to the center of **Earth** by looping the braids around a boulder or large crystal. Send any negative energy into the earth to be transmuted. Leave the ties in place.
• Now, using the same method, tie all 13 chakras to the **Moon**. This will connect you cosmically with the silver feminine energy of Creation. Leave this connection in place.
• Next, tie all 13 chakras to the **Sun**. This will connect you cosmically with the masculine energy of Creation. Leave this connection in place.

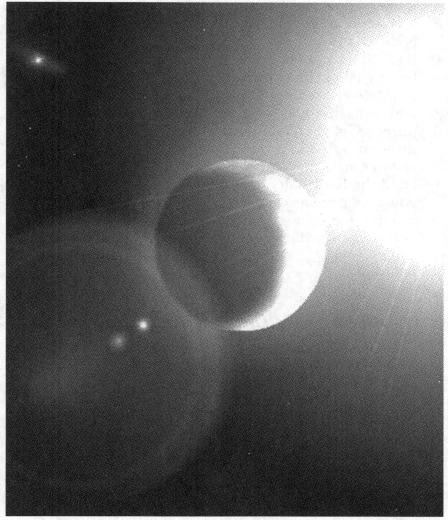

John Mason

- Feel the incredible power associated with these connections. Allow the unconditional Love and radiant Light to surround your auric field and permeate your four bodies.
- End this experience with your hands crossed at your heart chakra, imagine a blended ray consisting of the *gold*, *silver*, and *rose* rays. (This is a new triad of energy, one that just recently came to this planet for the purpose of environmental healing.) Have it flow through you and around you, then send it out to the rest of Earth.
- Hold the Earth, Moon, and Sun connections as long as you comfortably can. You can then consciously disconnect the braids, or just allow a natural disconnection--which will occur approximately 1/2 to 2 hours later.

Using the Double Infinity Symbol to Balance the Chakras

The *double infinity* symbol is the emblem for the 11th dimension (the dimension where many oversouls reside). The symbol appears as a horizontally laid figure eight, intersected by a vertically positioned figure eight. It resonates with a triad of energy composed of clear, violet, and rose rays.

Purpose: To connect in a conscious manner to your Oversoul; to embrace the state of oneness, knowledge, and empowerment that connection provides.

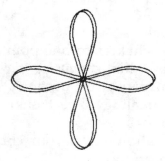

Procedure:
- Balance your chakras by turning them 13 times in each direction.
- Psychically, place the double infinity sign in each chakra, starting at the base.
- Within your mind's eye, trace the double infinity symbol one revolution horizontally along the figure eight, then one revolution vertically. Do this 13 times for each chakra.

NOTE: A variation of this technique is to place the double infinity symbol in only one chakras with the intent that it will automatically balance them all. This is a quick version of the above technique; apply it only when there is a time limitation.

Combining Chakras

Purpose: To create an energy field that is pure, compacted, and strong. *Combined chakras* have all of the rays, universes, and planets in one space, constituting an extension of Creation or Infinity Itself. At this level, whatever you wish for will manifest.

Procedure:
- Balance your chakras.
- Move all of your chakras to one point, usually the base or crown; this is called *collapsing the chakras*.
- From that point of power, accomplish whatever you wish. Perform healing, direct energy, manifest your deepest personal desires.
- When finished, allow all of your chakras to return to their original location.

Facilitating Communication

Purpose: To enhance communication between people by showing them the common link they share with each other. This exercise is to be done with a partner or with a group of people.

Procedure:
Note: All participants do this at the same time.
- Link your crown chakra, third eye, and heart chakras to the Moon.
- Link your throat and spleen chakras to the Sun.
- Link your solar plexus and base chakras to Earth.
- Collectively tie all of the chakras to each other. In other words, tie <u>your</u> crown chakra to your partner's crown chakra, or tie it to your neighbor's crown chakra, and so forth.
- Keep the chakras collectively linked for approximately one minute, then disconnect.
- Run violet energy through all of your chakras, turning each one that color. Then, spin each chakra three times to the left and three times to the right.

- Finally, change your chakras back to their normal colors. Spin each chakra three times to the left, and three times to the right.
- Re-ground and clear.

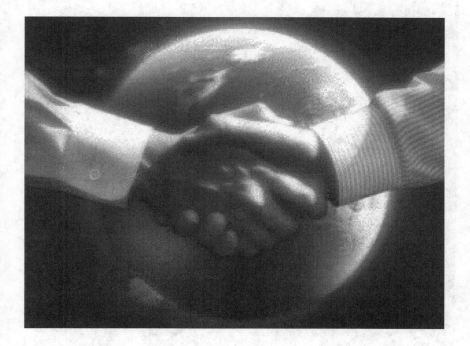

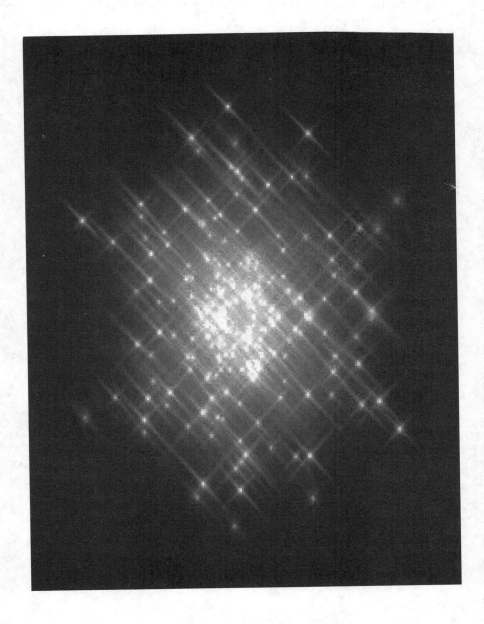

Chapter 21

The Black Ray Energy

"There is nothing either good or bad but thinking makes it so."

---William Shakespeare

Energy of the Tao

The black ray energy surrounds most of space. It also surrounds us. Although, it may not appear visually black, it is there nevertheless.

Black ray energy is contained within each of the elements: air, earth, fire, water, and ether; nothing in Creation can be separated from it.

Air appears colorless and tasteless, yet it carries the black ray at the atomic level.

Earth is filled with the black ray because it was the generator of the planet. The black ray is capable of manifesting a solid out of something intangible; the process is similar to the one used by Indian fakirs when they manifest a gemstone from thin air.

Fire's power is similar to the power of the black ray. When running the black ray, both healer and client feel "heated up".

Water is often used as a symbol of blessing and triumph. In great depths of water the color becomes black. Some people are comforted by water, others are fearful. The black ray permeates our oceans to varying degrees.

Ether, when concentrated, is black ray energy. Source or Spirit contains <u>all</u> of the rainbow colors, as does the color black.

As I stated in Chapter 16, you have nothing to fear from the black ray. It is a ray that contains all of the other rainbow rays; that is a sacred fact not an evil one. The black ray is very powerful, because it contains all of the movement and testing energy of the Cosmos.

Even today, the black ray is feared by those who don't understand it; there is prejudice, even by metaphysicians whose work I respect. Their views regarding the black ray seem to come from a fearful state, or one of ignorance. I wonder how many of these people have truly worked with this divine energy. Perhaps they are simply repeating the parrot-like propaganda of the Dark Ages. I know that I am inviting vehement opposition when I encourage the naysayers to work with the black ray without fear just once; they will undoubtedly see the unmistakable value it offers us all.

The black ray expeditiously cuts through any kind of resistance. Resistance is a closed web that prevents healing. Fear is the armor. By adding the black ray to the healing process, either by itself or activating it within the other rays, all fear and resistance fall by the wayside.

The common misconception of the black ray is that it facilitates a "black magician's" or sorcerer's tool of evil. This type of practitioner is <u>not</u> using a specific color, black or otherwise, but is consciously, magically manipulating the five elements for control and ill-gain.

Jesus' disciples were healers that utilized Spirit to heal. Simon Magus (not the apostle, Simon Peter) tried to buy magical power. He approached Peter and the other disciples in an attempt to purchase what they "had". They unanimously rebuked him, gently explaining that one could not buy Spirit; powerful energy comes from one's own willingness to live spiritually. Eventually, Simon did attain a kind of power, and proceeded to use it as a black magician. His misuse allowed his "power" to grow stronger*, whereby he frequently abused his neighbors. Eventually, Simon held the town in terror. Finally, his abusive power led to his death. Peter prayed to God that Simon's deception be stopped. Simon fell to his death while levitating above the Roman Forum in a challenge to Peter!

When you <u>wisely</u> practice color energy healing, you use the five elements as well as the rainbow color rays.

---

* This is due to the focused concentration of energy, albeit negative.

You always have access to the rays. If you spiritually work with color, as you evolve you can eventually create planets and universes, such is the power found in the 13 rainbow rays! Nicola Tesla knew it. Albert Einstein understood it. Paracelsus, the Renaissance Age alchemist physician, practiced it.

The Black Ray Guardians

A guardian of the black ray can be found inside each of the other rainbow color rays, including the black ray itself. For a multitude of reasons, Creation arranged for each color ray to contain the essence of the black ray. The primary focus of this decision was for transmutation, transformation, prevention of stagnation or movement, testing, and grounding.

The following names of the guardians of the black ray represent the English language vibration for their energy. In reality, they have no names at the twelfth dimension. You may use their names or not; it doesn't matter to them. You may for example, just call on the "black ray guardian within the red ray," and you will gain your results.

The following list of "names" includes the specialized purpose that each guardian has embraced within its appointed color ray.

Color	Ray Guardian and Purpose
Red	*Razalon* transforms the cellular part of the physical structure
Orange	*Auglia* transforms the creative part of the physical structure
Yellow	*Yachcta* transforms the power and energy at a physical level
Green	*Gossamer* transforms healing in general
Rose	*Alumina* transforms emotional healing
Translucent Blue	*Tartasnla* is for communication transmutation
Indigo	*Montage* is for mental transformation and for causal plane clearing
Violet	*Valurnia* is for intuition transformation and Akashic Record reading
Silver	*Aussylindiscara* is the female energy associated with facilitating intuition and psychic gifts
Gold	*Absalom a'Diem Abrianna et Abriella or "Goldie"* is a masculine energy for facilitating movement on all levels
White	*Lumina* is for providing protection
Clear	*Alpha* is for bringing forth truth and clarity
Black	*Omega or "Blackie"* is for bringing forth testing

The Black Ray Overlay Technique

Purpose: To practice concentration while utilizing the black ray in everything.

- This technique involves three people (the power of the triad). *A person running the black ray is like a laser beam.*
- Mentally link up together. This can be done with a chakra braiding, or simply a common intent. (Three

people running the black ray create a beam of light energy the size of a large spotlight.)

• Apply this intensified energy to your healing work; this kind of technique is to be used for entrenched cases of resistance where massive movement is needed for transmutation.

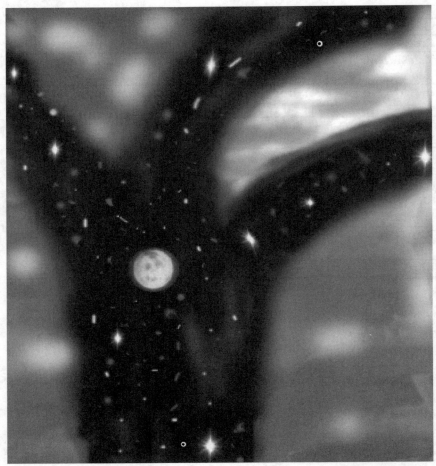

Sarah Steinbach

Chapter 22

Our Multidimensional Aspects

═══════════════════════════

"Man's a microcosm, or a little world, because he is an extract from all the stars and planets of the whole firmament, from the earth and the elements; and so he is their quintessence."

Theophrastus Paracelsus
Swiss Alchemist of the 16th century

243

Solar System Chakra Balancing

Purpose: To bring the solar system into our chakra system. Doing this serves the following purposes:
1. It facilitates our movement out into the world;
2. It enables us to have a stronger and more complete sense of who we are;
3. It clarifies and strengthens our sense of mission;
4. It moves us into a state of oneness with ourselves and all that is around us; and
5. It allows us to become aware of and embrace our God-like nature. *With this totality comes a realization that all that happens in our lives is of a synergistic nature. We are both the cause and the effect.*

Procedure:
- Using the following chart, picture the corresponding planet with the appropriate chakra and its color, starting with your base chakra.
- Spin the planet 13 times in each direction at your chakra.
- Continue up the chakra system until you have spun each chakra and its planet.

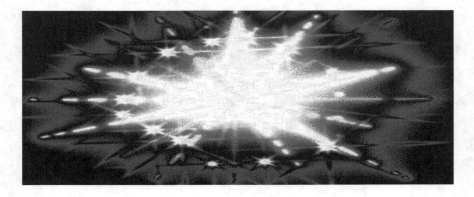

Chakra	Planetary Body	Element
Red	Sun	Fire
Orange	Moon	Fire/Earth
Yellow	Mercury	Fire/Earth
Green	Earth	Earth
Rose	Venus	Ether
Translucent Blue	Mars	Air
Indigo	Maldek *(Asteroid Belt)	Water
Purple	Jupiter	Ether
Silver	Saturn	Earth
Gold	Uranus	Ether
White	Neptune	Air
Clear	Pluto	Water
Black	Chiron†	All 5

Multidimensional Chakra Linking

Purpose: To expand your boundaries of knowledge, empowerment, psychic perception, and connection to all life-forms.

Procedure:
- Connect your chakras to the Earth, Sun, and Moon. (As explained in Chapter 20)
- Combine your chakras into one spot, either at the base or the crown. (Also explained in Chapter 20)
- From that point, send all 13 rays out to the *1st dimension*. The symbol of this dimension is the **cross**; the

---

* My guides tell me that the asteroid belt was originally a planet named Maldek. The planet's inhabitants were technologically unbalanced (not unlike Earth at the present time, if we continue on our foolhardy path) and blew-up their planet, creating the asteroid belt.

† A planetoid orbiting between Saturn and Uranus, discovered in 1977.

color triad is the *red*, *orange*, and *yellow* rays. The energy of this dimension is composed of the elements: air, water, fire, and earth. (You may hold this connective link throughout this technique)

- Next, send all 13 rays to the **2nd dimension**. The symbol of this dimension is the **medicine wheel**; the color triad is the *orange*, *yellow*, and *green* rays, and the energy of this dimension is the devic kingdom.

- Now, send all 13 rays to the **3rd dimension**. The symbol of this dimension is the **triangle**; the color triad is the *green*, *rose*, and *translucent blue* rays. The energy of this dimension is very physical consisting of many lifeforms, including human.

- Send all 13 rays to the **4th dimension**. The symbol of this dimension is the **5-pointed star**; the color triad is the *translucent blue*, *indigo*, and *violet* rays. The energy of this dimension is still physical, but at a less dense vibratory rate than the 3rd.

- Next, connect all 13 rays to the **5th dimension**. The symbol of this dimension is the **circle**; the color triad is the *violet*, *silver*, and *gold* rays. The energy of this dimension is even less dense than the 4th, with the beings appearing more translucent-looking.

- Now, connect all 13 rays to the **6th dimension**. The symbol of this dimension is the **diamond**; the color triad is the *gold*, *white*, and *clear* rays. The energy of this dimension is borderline non-physical; it is the transitional point between the physical and the non-physical. The beings on the 6th level are light forms.

- Send all 13 rays to the **7th dimension**. The symbol of this dimension is the **spiral**; the color triad is the *black*, *silver*, and *gold* rays. The energy of this dimension is non-physical; the beings are androgynously connected but still somewhat differentiated.

- Now, send all 13 rays to the **8th dimension**. The symbol of this dimension is the **octahedron**, or an eight-sided crystal. The color triad is the *silver*, *green*, and *red* rays. The energy of this dimension is non-physical; the beings are angelic with the light more blended. The guardians of the planets reside here.

- Next, send all 13 rays to the **9th dimension**. The symbol of this dimension is the **circle** with the **triangle** within it and the **square** within the triangle. The color triad is the *gold*, *translucent blue*, and *orange* rays. The energy of this dimension is still non-physical with less differentiation of the light. The guardians of the universes reside here.
- Send all 13 rays to the **10th dimension**. The symbol of this dimension is the **cadeusus**; the color triad is the *white*, *indigo*, and *yellow* rays. The energy of this dimension is the Radiant One.
- Next, connect all 13 rays to the **11th dimension**. The symbol of this dimension is the **double infinity** symbol; the color triad is the *clear*, *violet*, and *rose* rays. The energy of this dimension houses many of the oversouls, and is etheric.
- Now, connect all 13 rays to the **12th dimension**. The symbol of this dimension is the **dodecahedron**, the 12-sided crystal. The color triad is the *clear*, *white*, and *black* rays. The energy of this dimension is made up of pure color rays, or what is known as the guardians of the rays. It is an etic dimension.
- Send all 13 rays to the **13th dimension**. The symbol of this dimension is the **thousand-petaled lotus**; the color triad is the *black*, *clear*, and *white* rays. The energy of this dimension is the Source. It contains all elements, qualities, thoughts, etc.. It is an etheric dimension, and has no past or future, just the present.
- Finally, disconnect all of the 13 rays from the different dimensions. Bring your chakras back to their original locations. You may hold the connective links to the Earth, Sun, and Moon, or disconnect at this time.

- If you feel you need to ground again, do so. Remember that you are already linked to Earth, and that all of the braids will fade in a short while.

Connecting With Different Universes

Purpose: To expand your connection to others, to increase your power, and to amplify your energy and healing ability.

Procedure:
- Contained within each chakra is a universe; each universe is predominantly one color.
- Balance each of your chakras.
- Link your *base chakra* to the **red** universe. Don't be concerned if you don't know its exact location. Remember, that it is your <u>intent</u> that will help you intuitively link to the correct energy or location.
- Envision that universe. Allow for any perceptions to be seen, felt, heard, or known.
- Next, link the *spleen chakra* to the **orange** universe.
- Continue to connect your chakras to the associated universes. Eventually, you will be linked to each color universe.
- When completed, dissipate the energy. Re-ground.

The Out-of-Body Experience

How To Leave Your Body Consciously and Safely

Purpose: To meet your guides and teachers, to connect with other worlds and dimensions, and to increase your intuitive perceptions while connecting with other aspects of yourself.

This technique allows you to exit and re-enter your body through your heart chakra. This way of leaving your body is gentler than the standard "approach" of coming and going through your crown chakra. There is less of a chance for what we call "rocky" landings while using the heart chakra for out-of-body travel.

Procedure:
- Call forth the angels of the four corners (Michael, Gabriel, Ariel, Uriel) for protection.
- Balance your chakras by turning them 13 times in each direction.
- Bring *violet* energy down through your crown chakra to your base chakra.
- Turn the base chakra from red to violet. Then, turn the spleen chakra from orange to violet, and so forth up the chakra system.
- When you get to the crown chakra, add more violet to the violet already there. This will create a violet tornado or vortex around your head area.
- Bring the *silver* ray up from Mother Earth through your feet chakras. Allow the ray to spiral up through your body counter-clockwise.

- Bring the *gold* ray of Creation through your crown chakra. Spiral it down through your body in a clockwise manner.

- Eventually, have both rays meet at the *rose* part of your heart chakra. Feel your system as it is held in balance by the divine male and female energies.

- Visualize a portal (a rose colored doorway in the middle) where the silver and gold energies meet.

- Open the doorway and step through. Your essence should feel lighter, your body heavier.

- Travel to your destination.* Use your psychic perception abilities. Tell yourself you will remember when you bring the information found in this experience back.

- When it is time to return, travel back through the rose colored doorway at the heart chakra.

- Dissipate all excess gold and silver energy into the earth for healing purposes. Change all your chakras back to their original colors, starting at the crown and moving to the base.

- Ground, and re-balance your chakras.

---

* Destinations are infinite in variety. Some popular choices are different planes or planetary systems. Perhaps you've always yearned to see what 5th plane Neptune is like. This would be an interesting destination for you.

The Hyperspace Experience

Throughout the centuries, physics and metaphysics have been at odds, never finding a commonality. Many in the New Age movement assume that science doesn't accept anything that it can't explain and document repeatedly. The common scientific view is: if it isn't contained within a proven theorem, it isn't valid. Science has often relegated metaphysical thought and experience to the realm of fantasy and wishful thinking.

The "new physics" sounds suspiciously like metaphysics. Quantum theory embraces the concept of parallel universes, wormholes, space and time anomalies, and the idea that people create their own realities with their thoughts. What is science coming to!? I guess it was just a matter of "time" before the two apparent polar opposites (metaphysics and science) would meet in a common, acceptable middle.

Students of both physics and metaphysics say that we need to examine the nature of reality. For a long time now, modern society has held the belief that the environment impacts us; our collective consciousness has agreed to this particular reality. Quantum physics is now saying that we impact the environment; we do this by creating our own reality, with every single thought we think, every micro-second of the day.

Parallel Universes

Many science fiction writers and TV programs, such as <u>Star Trek</u>, have focused on the subject of parallel universes.

A *parallel universe*, or parallel planet, contains the same lifeforms as does its parallel counterpart, but it is the antithesis of the other. It is a mirror image, though it may look and feel autonomous with its own, separate value system. Your "double" (or even "evil" twin) may truly reside in the Earth's parallel universe.

Not every universe or planet has a reflection; the parallel universe is a twin, not a shadow.

A planet in Parallel Universe #1 cannot see its counterpart in Parallel Universe #2. A planet in Parallel Universe #2 cannot see its counterpart in Parallel Universe #1. However, in the wormhole that connects the two, you would be able to see both, simultaneously.

Exercise: Traveling to a Parallel Universe
- Balance your chakras. Collapse them to either the base or the crown chakra. Send a link into the Earth, Sun, and Moon.
- Send out a chakra link (consisting of the 13 rays) to our neighboring parallel universe (located on the dark side of the Moon).
- Allow your consciousness to travel to this parallel universe. Find it's "Earth".
- Use your strongest psychic gifts (see, feel, hear, or know) to perceive the energy of Earth's twin.
- After a few minutes, bring your attention back to your present reality. **Be sure to dissipate the chakra link.**
- As always, clear and ground. Re-balance your chakra system.

Three other ways to travel to a parallel universe:
1. Find a wormhole   (The technique for entering the wormhole is described later in this chapter.)
2. Find a black hole. (The technique for entering a black hole is described later in this chapter.)
3. Find a "lightbridge". This is an etheric or non-physical energy bridge which is accessed on Earth. It is generally found in places wherein there is an emotional attachment or meaning--such as a birthplace, current home, loved ones' home, sacred place, and so forth.

Pulsars

A *pulsar* is formed from neutron stars[*] rotating around each other in an opposing dance of attraction and repulsion. Huge amounts of heat and light are generated by a pulsar, along with strong, intense surges of gravity and magnetism. Light waves, radio waves, and radar bombard the pulsar's stars. All of the color rays, including the alchemical colors, are present in a concentrated array. By traveling out-of-body to these pulsar stars, one gains a sense of balance.

The beings on these stars are more visual and have more amplified psychic powers. They also have a better sense of protective defense mechanisms. To temporarily visit one of these space amusement parks, use the following technique:
• Balance your chakras. Do the double infinity technique as described in Chapter 20.

---

[*] A *neutron star* is formed from a burned out core of a massive star which collapses down into a very dense, small (typically 20 mile diameter) mass of incredibly strong magnetic field.

- Travel out-of-body using the technique mentioned earlier in this chapter.
- Focus your intent as you locate one of the pulsars within our own galaxy. [There are several possibilities. A good choice would be the "young" 900 year old Crab Pulsar, located in the center of the Crab Nebula in the constellation of Taurus, 6500 light years away from Earth.]
- Look for a planet, within the pulsar, that contains water and lifeforms.
- Compact all of your chakras at your heart center.
- From your heart chakra, send a large braid consisting of the 13 color rays to the pulsar.
- Through your heart link, begin to perceive and investigate the neutron star.
- After a few minutes, travel back along the braid to your body. Re-enter your body through your heart chakra.
- Dissipate the color braid.
- Clear and ground. Re-balance your chakras.

Quasars

A *quasar* is a galaxy with the luminescence of a hundred galaxies. It is the birth of a galaxy and the beginnings of a new universe.

Purpose: To help you regain your energy when you are feeling "run down", or needing to specifically send healing to a particular body part. Quasars normalize the body to its correct frequency wave.

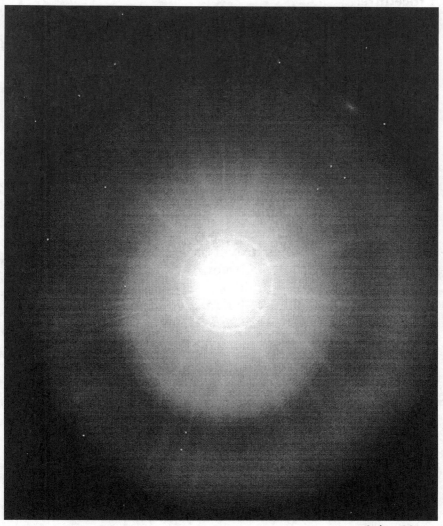

John Mason

Procedure:

- Ground and protect yourself.
- Balance your chakras. Collapse them to one of your chakra points (base or crown).
- Have the universe build you a "quasar filter" to shield you from the overpowering radio waves emitted by the quasar. It will convert the radio waves to color or other forms of energy that the human body can tolerate.
- Send out a braided link consisting of the 13 color rays to the quasar.
- The radio waves emitted by the quasar are transformed through your shield into color and other energy. Allow this light to fill your body, balancing it.
- After a few minutes, travel back along the braid to your body. Come in through your heart chakra.
- Dissipate the color braid.
- Clear and ground. Re-balance your chakras.

Wormholes

Wormholes are a primitive set of highways connecting planetary bodies, or parallel universes. Generally they do not shift, contrary to many science fiction plot lines. Some are invisible while others are visible. The uninitiated, without the knowledge and understanding of the wormhole, could cross its walls without realizing that it's there. No damage is incurred by this on either side; the wormhole, as well as the traveler, remain unaltered. The wormhole is a self-healing structure.

Finding an entrance to a wormhole enables one to travel from point A to point B in a relatively short time, even if the two points are thousands of light-years away from each other. The wormhole can be natural or man made. They are undetectable with 3rd plane instrumentation.

Wormholes alter the time/space continuum.

Exercise: Entering and Traveling Through the Wormhole
- Balance your chakras. Collapse them to one of your chakra points (base or crown).
- Send out a braided link consisting of the 13 color rays to the nearest wormhole. [It is a "man-made" wormhole that connects Earth and Venus.]
- Psychically follow your chakra link to the wormhole entrance.
- Little by little, allow yourself to go into the wormhole. Experience the wormhole by using your strongest psychic senses.

  NOTE: You will find that the wormhole literally looks like the inside of a worm; it is ridged and is tan in color.
- After a short time, follow your chakra link back to your chakra point. Unlink your chakra connection.
- Clear and ground. Re-balance your chakras.

Time Travel

New Age mystics tell us that time* is speeding up, not only for individuals but for Earth as a planetary body. This has created a quickening of the Earth's vibrational rate, resulting in massive clearings for both people and the planet. As we personally and collectively purge our toxic bodies, we can begin to embrace certain concepts relating to the time/space continuum, ideas that were beyond our comprehension during prior periods of limited, linear consciousness.

The concept of time travel is an age-old intriguing precept, one that has seemed to lurk outside the realm of possibility. However, history is filled with verifiable, logic defying stories of people who suddenly disappear from sight, as though they entered some sort of time/space warp.

Many ordinary people have experienced "instantaneity"; while riding in their cars they find that they have traveled certain distances in too short of a time span (an hour trip has taken only 1/2 hour, for example). Similarly, they might end up far from their planned destination knowing that it was impossible to have navigated such a distance in the time elapsed. I, myself, have had several experiences of this kind. This usually happens while I'm on a spiritual quest of some sort, or in a particularly spiritual state of mind. When this phenomenon oc-

---

* Time is an artificial measurement, used to calculate the movements of planets and to record events. True time is not linear or monochronic; it is a continuous circle, or spiral, and it is polychronic in nature. True time encompasses parallel lifetimes and universes. Decades within these worlds can be compared to leaves on a tree; a tree whose branches lead to one's life path or direction.

curs, we have somehow warped time, by being willing to think holographically instead of linearly.

On the other dimensions, time travel is an accepted, normal and common occurrence. When 3rd plane embodied humans are ready, the physical act of time travel will occur naturally. Throughout history, in different parts of our world, there have been some individuals who have understood the fluidity of time, the manipulation of matter and energy, and the validity of the holographic self. Time travel will unfold naturally on Earth when our complete understanding and subsequent spiritual alignment is in place. This will probably not occur until we, as a species, achieve a less-dense planetary consciousness.

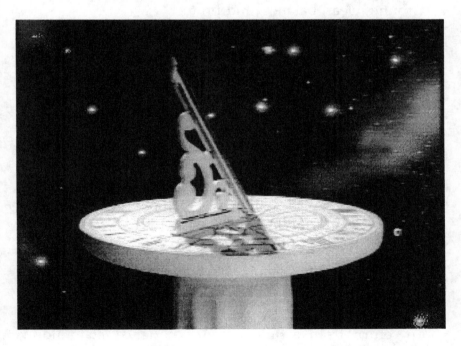

Time Travel -- Stage 1

Purpose: To acquaint you with the fundamental laws needed to initiate the time travel experience. These involve *only* the emotional, mental, and spiritual bodies at this level, *not* the physical body. (It is similar to an out-of-body experience.) As with all techniques explained in this book, practice is imperative for adeptness.

Procedure:
• First of all, choose a safe place, and then determine where you will go. Make it simple. Select a time period that interests you.
• Ground, clear, balance, and protect.
• Make a concoction of geranium, rose, and violet flower essences (essential oils) to facilitate your experience. Lightly, apply the fragrant oil under your nose.
• Connect your chakras into the Earth, Sun, and Moon.
• Link your chakras to each of the dimensions.
• Bring forth a triad of energies involving the *rose*, the *indigo*, and the *violet*.
• Locate the thymus, the pituitary, and the pineal glands in your body.
• Unite the three glands with each other (in a triangle shape) by connecting the braid of the rose, indigo, and violet rays and linking the braid between them.
• Now, bring forth the *black* ray, and send it through the braid to activate movement.
• Hold the intent of your destination firmly in place. Allow the executed "hook-up" to move you into a space of receptivity to the experience.
• To return from a time travel experience, state aloud, "Present reality now," or have a facilitator say it aloud to you.

- Dissipate the braids. Ground, clear, balance, and protect yourself again.

Note: Realize that time travel is a very special ability; it may take repeated practice before it becomes a comprehensible experience. While learning, you may actually experience aspects of time travel that you're not even aware of. However, you may not be clear about what you are seeing or feeling, similar to the out-of-body state.

Traveling Into Black Holes and White Holes

Black holes are collapsed stars. Since no light can escape from the star's enormous gravitational field, the collapsed star becomes black in color. Science tells us that the density of a black hole is so large that light is forced to orbit around it. There is a "point of no return" that surrounds a black hole. Scientists believe that there are tens of millions of black holes in our Milky Way galaxy alone.

On the cutting edge, modern physics postulates that black holes may be gateways to an alternative universe, even a "mirror" or parallel universe. There is much speculation regarding the theory that black holes may be openings to rips in the fabric of time. Those of us who have psychically traveled into and out of these black holes know these speculations to be a reality.

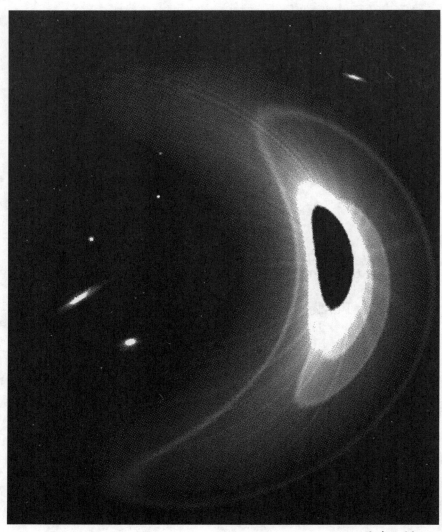

John Mason

White holes are frequently found on the other side of black holes. They join together, much like a chalice, with the center point being a place of balanced gravitational pull. The white hole itself has a propulsion effect, a kind of reverse gravity. It is a black hole running backward in time.

So, what would be the purpose of psychically traveling into black and white holes?

Purpose: To activate the kundalini. To help you attune yourself with the lower chakras, to create movement and processing, and clean out unnecessary energy debris. You can do this exercise individually, or with a group.

Procedure:
- Balance your chakras.
- Connect your chakras to the Earth, the Sun, and the Moon. (See Chapter 20 for the technique.)
- Do the "Solar System Balancing" technique as described earlier in this chapter.
- Now, bring the double infinity sign into each of your chakras. (See Chapter 20 for the technique)
- Combine your chakras at a single point (at either the crown or the base).
- Send the chakra link to the middle point of the *black hole* (e.g., you can visualize the one in the constellation of Virgo).
- Feel yourself being pulled into the vortex.
- Experience the black hole. Use all of your psychic senses. What you experience will be unique to you. There is incredible light, sound, and movement within the black hole.

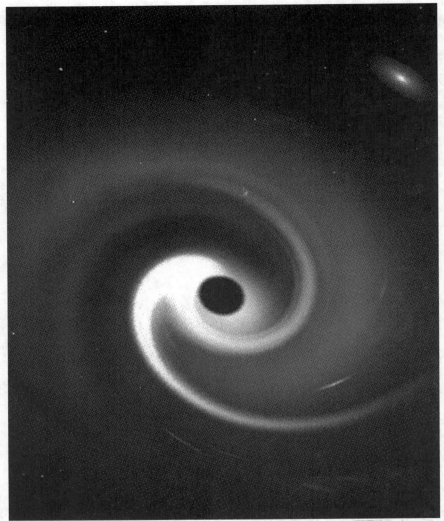

John Mason

- Allow yourself to be drawn towards the middle of the hole and compressed down.
- You'll find yourself in a place of perfect time/space balance, or E=M=C (energy=matter=consciousness).
- Stay there for a few minutes.
- Now, begin to feel yourself being drawn into the *white hole* on the other side.
- As you integrate with the white hole, feel yourself become it.
- Let the white hole propel you out of its center at seven times the speed of light.
- Come back into your body. Clear, ground, and re-balance your chakras.

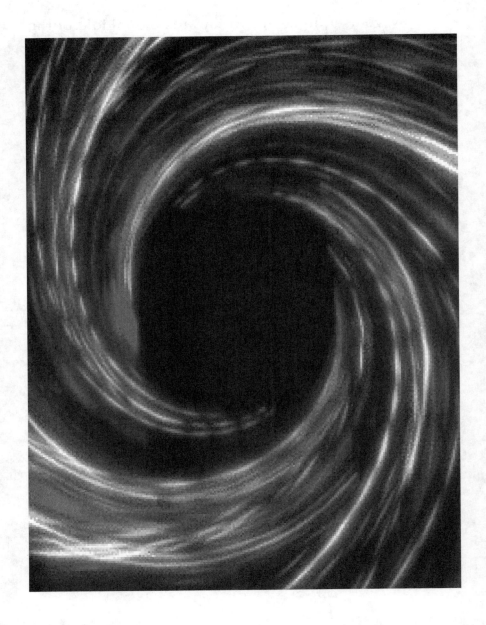

Chapter 23

Facing our Shadow

"If you gaze for long into the abyss, the abyss gazes into you."

--- *Nietzsche*

The Shadow Self

Through the process of healing ourselves and others, we bring more light into our physical, mental, and emotional bodies. This light is composed of higher vibrational energies; these energies show us aspects of ourselves that we have been inclined to disown, project onto others, or completely repress. These darker aspects of our personality comprise our *shadow self*.

To become whole and optimize your healing capabilities, it is important for each one of us to embrace our shadow self. This includes the shadow self's feelings and capabilities that we have placed in "exile". For different people, in different families and cultures, what is acceptable and unacceptable varies. For example, some families permit anger to be openly expressed, others do not. Some permit open expression of sexuality, vulnerability, and strong emotions...others do not. Values also vary; importance may be placed upon material acquisition, intellectual development, artistic expression, or traditional religious beliefs. This kind of variety really does "make the world go 'round!".

In literature, the most famous example of the shadow self can be found in the story of Dr. Jekyl and Mr. Hyde by Robert Louis Stevenson. In the grim tale, a male character is pursued for a crime he's accused of committing. In desperation, he swallows a powder and undergoes a dramatic change in character, a transformation so drastic that he is unrecognizable. The kind, hard working scientist known as Dr. Jekyl is transformed into the violent and relentless Mr. Hyde, a man whose evil takes on greater, darker significance as the dream story unfolds.

We must integrate such exiled parts of ourselves; dark, fragmented bits of our personality that have been split off from our consciousness, to become more whole and complete. When we repress, deny, and project internal impulses onto the external landscape, we unknowingly disempower ourselves. We create the illusion that we are being victimized by forces outside ourselves, perpetuating the belief that we have little or no control over our lives.

If we assume that everything and everyone is interconnected and interrelated, we have the capability to determine our relationship to every person or situation that we face. In other words, we decide to **respond** instead of **react**.

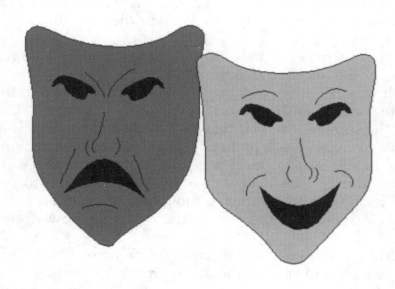

Multidimensional Chakra Linking to the Shadow Dimensions--14 through 23

During the creation of the 13 dimensions, initially unbeknownst to the Creator and the rest of the Universe, the *shadow dimensions* began to appear. This grouping formed a parallelism, a kind of <u>Alice Through the Looking Glass</u>.

The original 13 dimensions that were created from the Void by the Creator had a certain substantial quality which contained color vibration. The existence of the shadow dimensions was not immediately apparent to the Source. It was a lovely surprise to God, and He/She decided to allow us all the opportunity to discover the new creation for ourselves.

These shadow planes are <u>reflections</u> and are energetically of the negative (feminine) polarity.

It was incredibly exciting to receive the knowledge that there were other dimensions beyond the original 13! During the summer of 1994, two colleagues and I took out-of-body voyages to each of them. I then passed this information to my master level students, as we journeyed together during class. I now pass this knowledge on to you, to stretch your boundaries of thought and experience, and acquaint you with the newly discovered shadow dimensions.

This multidimensional view offers us one more way to "clear" and an additional approach to healing. Remember, as with any technique, it takes practice to fully perceive and master. Again, as with any exercise in this book, perceive the difference with your strongest psychic sense.

- Balance your chakras. Then connect them to the Earth, Sun, and Moon. (See Chapter 20)
- Now, combine your chakras to one spot, either the base or the crown. (See Chapter 20)
  Note: The triads of alchemical color rays may create a color that's a bit unexpected. In some cases, certain rays of the triad may be dominant, or in a greater concentration, over the others.
- Send all 13 rays from that chakra point to the *14th dimension*. This plane appears soft and feminine, primordial-like. It is a place of perfect balance, wherein yin and yang are in absolute harmony. This is the first "shadow universe". The alchemical color triad of energy which created this plane is the *black, white,* and *clear*, forming a **gray** color. This dimension's symbol is the **yin-yang**.
- Unlink your chakra connection to the 14th dimension and link-up to the *15th dimension*. This plane houses liquid beings (ocean-like; similar to the aliens in the movie The Abyss), semi-solid, jelly-like, and translucent. The energy focus is laser-like; it is the flip side to the sprite and fairy kingdoms. The alchemical color triad of energy which created this dimension is the *gold, silver,* and *white,* forming a **light silvery gold** color. The symbol for this dimension is an **hourglass**.
- Unlink your chakra connection to the 15th dimension and link-up to the *16th dimension*. This plane is composed of very refined energy; there is a lot of precision here. In is inhabited by animals now extinct on Earth. The atmosphere is composed of 100% oxygen. The alchemical color triad of energy which created this plane is the *green, translucent blue,* and *clear,* forming a **teal** color. This dimension's symbol is a **planet** that looks like Earth.
- Unlink your chakra connection to the 16th dimension and link-up to the *17th dimension*. This plane con-

271

tains Celtic energy; it is filled with the power of healing and the dynamic of ancient wisdom. Infinite wealth and abundance reside in this dimension where all desires are met. The alchemical color triad of energy which created this plane is the *emerald green, mint green,* and *white,* forming a **creamy jade green** (like a moss agate stone). The symbol is the **Celtic cross**.

- Unlink your chakra connection to the 17th dimension and link-up to the *18th dimension*. This plane appears to have very focused heart energy, a light and airy feeling. Crystalline structures can be utilized in a laser-like way. The alchemical color triad of energy which created this plane is the *white, black,* and *clear,* forming a **glossy black with white spots** (colored like a snowflake obsidian stone). Its symbol is a **feather**.

- Unlink your chakra connection to the 18th dimension and link-up to the *19th dimension*. This plane has American Indian energy. There is a powerful sense of "knowingness" and "beingness", spiritual strength, and speaking one's truth. The alchemical color triad of energy which created this dimension is the *translucent blue* (turquoise shade), *black,* and *red* (coral-shade), forming a **coral** color. Its symbol is the **arrowhead**.

- Unlink your chakra connection to the 19th dimension and link-up to the *20th dimension*. This plane contains mental energy, with no sense of an emotional dynamic. Here, one sees things from a great height. This level is a communication center. Within its atmosphere, there is a sense of swallowing and expanding. The alchemical color triad of energy which created this plane is the *indigo, green,* and *black* forming a **cobalt blue** color. The symbol for this dimension is a **circle containing a small circle within it** (similar to a donut).

- Unlink your chakra connection to the 20th dimension and link-up to the *21st dimension*. This plane is sub-

cle containing a small circle within it (similar to a do-nut).

- Unlink your chakra connection to the 20th dimension and link-up to the **21st dimension**. This plane is sub-stance-free; it is completely gaseous. It has no apparent surface area or dimension. The alchemical color triad of energy which created this dimension is the *clear, silver,* and *white,* forming a **silvery white** color. The symbol for this dimension is the true, **ancient Hopi swastika** (not the Nazi version, which was reversed).

- Unlink your chakra connection to the 21st dimension and link-up to the **22nd dimension**. This plane is also gaseous. It is very quixotic; things keep shifting and changing rapidly. The alchemical color triad of energy which created this plane is the *translucent blue, clear,* and *gold,* forming **bluish gold**. The symbol for this dimension is an **ocean wave**.

- Unlink your chakra connection to the 22nd dimension and link-up to the **23rd dimension**. This plane is a place of perfect alchemy. The alchemical color triad of energy which created this dimension is the *silver, gold,* and *clear,* forming a **goldish silver** color. The symbol for this dimension is a **diamond gem**.

- Unlink your chakra connection to the 23rd dimension. Make sure all of your chakras are clear of links to the various dimensions. If you wish to leave your chakras connected to the Earth, Sun, and Moon, do so. They will dissolve automatically after a short time.

- Bring your attention back to Earth. Allow your chakras to return to their normal position, and re-balance them.

- Ground.

Dimension	Symbol	Ray Colors
14th	Yin-Yang	Black, White, Clear
15th	Hourglass	Gold, Silver, White
16th	Earth-like planet	Gold, Silver, White
17th	Celtic Cross	Green, Blue, Clear
18th	Feather	Emerald Green, Moss Green, White
19th	Arrowhead	White, Black, Clear
20th	Circle inside a circle	Turquoise, Black, Coral Red
21st	Ancient Hopi swastika	Clear, Silver, White
22nd	Ocean Wave	Blue, Clear, Gold
23rd	Diamond face	Silver, Gold, Clear

This previous technique is only one way to enter the shadow dimensions, or any of the other dimensions. Another way to enter every dimension is to find a "keyhole"; each dimension has a portal or veil which separates it from the other dimensions. A keyhole is very small, and appears unstable as it energetically moves around a bit. If you can't find one to travel through, ask your guides for assistance. Still, another way is to find a black hole; this will usually toss you into an unspecified plane. To get back to the 3rd dimension, just state your intent. Do not fear you won't find your way home. Even falling asleep will bring you back.

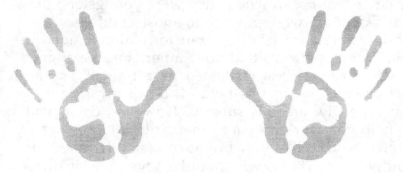

Integrating Your Inner Child

Children generally understand (better than adults) how the healing process works. Unless there has been great trauma, children simply have fewer blocks, more openness to bringing their bodies back to a state of health. Children carry a greater acceptance of multiple realities. They don't question, as adults usually do, that we are capable of multidimensionality, many levels of consciousness. Often, they carry memories of other dimensional experiences.

Jesus said that unless you become as a child, you shall not enter into the kingdom of heaven. *This is a very important point.*

Today, integrating your *inner child* is a very popular therapeutic method. People are obviously beginning to realize that they have become fragmented beings by isolating, ignoring, or even abusing the "little child" within them. This fragmentation, whether mild or severe, leads to a myriad of adult dysfunctions, such as, difficulty feeling emotions, including joy or love. Some find it hard to relate to children; others carry abandonment and trust issues that are decades old. In severe cases, adults complete an ugly circle that began when they were youngsters; they are abused children who grow up to abuse children.

To fully experience healing, transformation, and illumination, it is imperative that your inner child be aligned within you. This is best facilitated by a trained psychotherapist or specialist in this field. It is not my intention to venture deeply into this subject. However, color healing can help you work on your inner child integration.

Children tend to like very bright colors such as red, orange, and yellow. That is why popular toys come in these colors. These bright colors generate a lot of energy and happiness for little kids.

On the other hand, most adults are drawn to muted pastels, or calming colors such as rose, green, and blue. Colors such as red, orange, or black may even frighten adults; these colors can be equated with danger, as in the case of red fire engines.

The average adult hides from his or her inner child. One way to connect with the child you were is to discover what color palette you enjoyed as a youngster. See if you can locate some old photographs of yourself wearing certain colors, or artwork you may have produced as a child.

child's palette, as well as, for your inner child to experience the adult's palette.

• Begin to use some of the child's colors. This might mean that you wear some of those colors, or that you surround your environment with decorative items colored with the old palette.

• By implementing your "inner child's" palette, many other cellular memories will come to the surface for rediscovery and self-integration.

Camouflaging Energy

The process of camouflaging energy involves tuning into an other's auric field, and then matching it in an energetic, color way. You do not need to match it in a vibrational manner (which is like their individual energy fingerprint), but simply in the color pattern. Your goal is to fool the receiver into thinking that your energy field is his or her <u>own</u> energy field.

Why do this at all? The answer includes ethical and unethical reasons.

The ethical reasons include using this camouflage technique as a process for facilitating healing, particularly when working with a resistant client. This assumes that he or she has given permission for the healing. The healer can then "match" the energy, facilitating healing. This process may be done in emergency healing involving a team of healers, as well.

The unethical reasons for camouflaging energy include "black magic" misuses of energy. *Unethical camouflaging of energy will accumulate negative karma for the doer*. Unethical reasons may range from being "nosey" about another person, to the desire to siphon off their energy field, for what is perceived as extra energy. In other words, the doer becomes an "energy vampire". Another immoral reason for camouflaging energy is to control another person for malevolent purposes.

The usual, recommended protective method of enclosing yourself in a chrome ball or lead shield has failed to protect against these camouflagers.

I recommend a **Teflon® shield**, with the outermost layer composed of *white*, the middle layer of *clear*, and the inside layer of *black*.

Some cases require the stronger measure of invoking a **cellular footprint**. It is a web placed around the one being attacked, composed of elemental crystals or gemstones to block the camouflager. To achieve a cellular footprint, ask the universe to set this energy grid into place. The angelic beings will immediately invoke this protection for you.

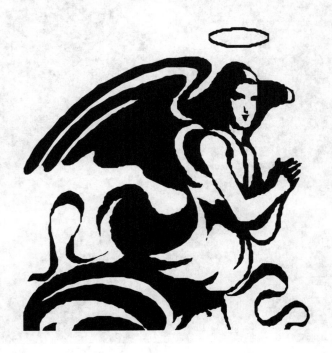

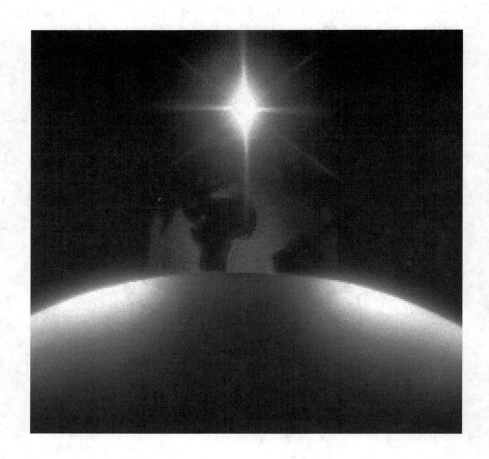

Chapter 24

Alchemy Made Easy

---

*"When you fix your heart
on one point, then nothing
is impossible for you."*

-- *Buddha*

Some of the most exciting, newer data I've channeled involves the connection between the glands and organs of the physical body, and the emotional, mental, and spiritual bodies. This is different than the holistic healing modality called <u>visceral work</u>*. That method involves tuning into the various organs of the body through touch, then determining the emotional messages they convey. It is excellent work, albeit incomplete because it involves only the emotional state of being, not the mental or spiritual components. From my understanding it also only works with the organs, not the glands. I present this new information to help expand and clarify the process of visceral work, to show that there is a direct correlation between the viscera and the mental and emotional states of imbalance. Additionally, I will show the viscera's connection to the psychic and spiritual gifts, and how to activate them for enlightenment.

To work with the organs and glands of the body, you need to know what their function is and where they are located. As part of my regular classes, I give my students a course in basic anatomy prior to working with this data. It is strongly suggested that you purchase a simple anatomy book, such as one of the anatomy coloring books, or a large, detailed anatomical drawing to refer to the specific viscera as they are mentioned.

Some people are missing a gland or organ; however, that doesn't mean they are missing that particular emotional trigger or psychic gift. The energy field of that gland or organ is usually still intact. Everyone has heard stories of amputees who lose a limb, yet still feel sensation in that part of the body; this is called *phantom pain*, an interest-

---

* It is interesting to note that the word *visceral* is secondarily defined as "intuitive or emotional feeling," implying that at some level people understand that the viscera of the human body reflect our feelings and psychic senses

ing physical phenomena. If a Kirlian photo were taken of that limb, one would still observe an energy field where the limb used to be. The energy or electromagnetic field is still present, even if the physical part is not. That specific section of the body still contains all emotional/mental memories and the potential for psychic activation. For example, I lost my appendix several years ago and yet, telepathy (the gift the appendix offers) is one of my stronger psychic traits.

For the next several techniques it is recommended that, as you work on a client, you do an initial body scan. Afterwards, you may focus on specific areas that catch your attention. When you locate a spot you wish to heal, run the specific color rays the visceral part requires. If you pick up emotional and mental imbalance, gently inform the client of your perceptions. Allow him/her to communicate any emotions or thoughts that come up at that time.

Emotional/Mental Imbalances of the Glands and Organs

Purpose: To get in touch with any areas relating to mental or emotional conflict or imbalance. To allow a calming, re-balancing healing to take place.

Gland/Organ	Dysfunctional Emotional/Mental Trait
Appendix	Can be shut down, not processing, or processing too much energy. Pain vs. pleasure center. Linked to the gallbladder.
Tonsils	Not wanting to feel. A state of fear. Fear vs. comfort. "Running away" vs. embracing something.

Gland/Organ	Dysfunctional Emotional/Mental Trait
Middle Ear	Not wanting to hear. Resistance vs. receptivity.
Adenoids	Standstill. Immobilization vs. fluidity.
Pineal	Not wanting to see. Blindness vs. perception.
Crown	Denial of self. Isolation, fragmentation, separation vs. wholeness.
Pituitary	Fragmentation of male and female energies. Fear of death and sense of finiteness. Stagnation vs. growth.
Hypothalamus	Feeling that the physical is all there is. Trying to control and manipulate the physical. Unconsciousness vs. consciousness.
Parathyroid	Male/female imbalance. The denigration of one and idealization of the other vs. balance in the male and female energies.
Thalamus	Unable to regulate a sense of good and evil vs. an awareness of the difference.
Thyroid	Illusion vs. truth (or pure intent).
Thymus	Lack of unconditional love, or love with expectations and judgments vs. unconditional love.
Adrenals	Fear of owning one's power. Paralyzing fear. Misuse of "fight or flight" response. The <u>Celestine Prophecy</u> control dramas vs. not playing control dramas.
Pancreas	Feeling unnurtured, a lack of sweetness in life vs. feeling nurtured and joyful.
Liver	Self-destruction vs. self-respect.
Spleen	Lack of creativity/power. Shutting down emotions or a center of anger, such as "venting one's spleen" vs. appropriate expression of emotion.

Gland/Organ	Dysfunctional Emotional/Mental Trait
Heart	Shutting down emotions. "Heartbreak" vs. appropriate expression of emotion and open heart chakra.
Lungs	Restriction to prana energy. Grief response vs. joyful and flowing energy.
Gonads/Uterus	Difficulty in generating life and/or love vs. expression and allowance of life and love.
Kidneys/Bladder	Shame, guilt. Can't process or filter toxic emotions vs. the ability to do so.
Large Intestine	Shame, blame vs. personal strength or "intestinal fortitude".
Small Intestine	Frustration of the emotional body. Unwillingness to listen to others vs. mental flexibility and emotional fluidity.
Stomach	Feeling unloved or rejected vs. making balanced judgments/discernments.

The Psychic/Spiritual Connections of the Glands and Organs

Balancing Only

Purpose: This technique is to balance the specific gland or organ in the spiritual and psychic areas. It is not meant to activate or trigger the trait, merely to balance.

Gland/ Organ	Trait	Color (Used To Balance Only)
Appendix	Telepathy	Turquoise
Tonsils	Clairsentience	Coral
Middle ear	Clairaudience	White
Adenoids	Telekinesis	Mustard yellow
Pineal	Clairvoyance	Rose
Crown	Godhead, All that is	Violet
Pituitary	Bridges physical with the non-physical bodies, especially when the masculine and feminine are merged. Physical immortality	Orange
Hypothalamus	Immortality/Spiritual	Indigo
Parathyroid	Related to the male/ female balance (yin/yang). Kundalini link	Mustard yellow
Thalamus	Spiritual center for connecting with other people.	Grey
Thyroid	Sacred OM vibration. Commitment to speaking cosmic truth.	Translucent Blue
Thymus	Portal of expression for unconditional love.	Black
Adrenals	Source of raw power. Related to shamanic healing.	Green
Pancreas	Sense of taste, sweet. Related to nurturing.	Sky blue

Gland/ Organ	Trait	Color (Used To Balance Only)
Liver	Visceral way of releasing anger. Detox center for processing toxic emotions. Related to self-love at a personal level.	Red
Spleen	Power plus creativity.	Green
Heart	Source of divine love.	Green/Rose
Lungs	Flow of prana energy	Rose
Gonads/Uterus	Linked to kundalini, bringing forth life, divine love.	Orange
Kidneys/ Bladder	Filtering system. Essential for purging.	Orange
Large Intestine	Absorption of ideas, spiritual clearing and cleansing.	White
Small Intestine	Assimilation and transformation	Clear
Stomach	Capacity to assimilate information and compartmentalize or discern (how one sizes up the world).	White

Psychically and Spiritually Activating the Glands and Organs

Purpose: This technique will activate, while allowing for a transformation, the psychic and spiritual abilities. As with any progressive, intensive technique, use it with wisdom. While working, always remain in a physically, emotionally, mentally, and spiritually balanced state for optimum empowerment.

Gland/ Organ	Trait	Color Used To Transform or Activate
Appendix	Telepathy	Red
Tonsils	Clairsentience	Translucent Blue
Middle ear	Clairaudience	Indigo
Adenoids	Telekinesis	Indigo
Pineal	Clairvoyance	Purple
Crown	Godhead, All that is	Gold
Pituitary	Bridges physical with the non-physical bodies, especially when the masculine and feminine are merged. Physical immortality	Indigo
Hypo-thalamus	Immortality/Spiritual	White
Parathyroid	Related to the male/female balance (yin/yang). Kundalini link	Rose, Translucent Blue
Thalamus	Spiritual center for connecting with people.	Silver, Green
Thyroid	Sacred OM vibration. Commitment to speaking cosmic truth	Translucent Blue
Thymus	Portal of expression for uncondi-tional love	Green, Rose

Gland/ Organ	Trait	Color Used To Transform or Activate
Adrenals	Source of raw power. Related to shamanic	Yellow to increase. Black to decrease.
Pancreas	Sense of taste, sweet. Related to nurturing	Rose
Liver	Visceral way of releasing anger. Detox center for processing toxic emotions. Related to self-love at a personal level	Green
Spleen	Power plus creativity	Orange
Heart	Source of divine love	Rose
Lungs	Inflow/outflow of prana energy	Green
Gonads/ Uterus	Linked to kundalini, bringing forth life, divine love	Orange
Kidneys/ Bladder	Filtering system. Essential for purging	Red
Large Intestine	Absorption of ideas, spiritual clearing and cleansing	Black, Clear
Small Intestine	Assimilation and transformation	Silver, Black, White
Stomach	Capacity to assimilate information and compartmentalize or discern (how one sizes up the world around oneself).	Blend of rose and green

Psychic Surgery

The following technique does not involve the physical penetration of the body by the practitioner (in the manner of the renowned psychic surgeons of the Philippines). Based on my study of traditional psychic surgeons, I believe that they have learned the art of alchemy, and the manipulation of elemental fire and water. They understand that the body is vibrating molecules; they have also learned the art of separating those molecules without pain and with minimal blood loss. When the surgery is complete, traditional psychic surgeons are able to seamlessly reconnect those molecules.

My technique is not dissimilar in its healing intent as it penetrates the physical body and its energy systems. The difference is that my method doesn't separate the physical molecular structure of the physical body. The "surgeon's" hands do not enter the patient's body cavities; however, the modality does allow energetic, healing penetration to impact all of the client's bodies.

Psychic Surgery Technique

Purpose: To instill movement (especially in tough cases) of "stuck" energy or major resistance by the client. To awaken him/her from the self-created illusion of sickness. To eliminate fear and bring perfect creation into being.

Using the hands to direct the energy provides extra stimulus.

Procedure:
- Link your chakras to the Earth, Sun, and Moon. (See Chapter 20)
- Next, link your chakras to each of the 13 dimensions. (See Chapter 22)

- Begin to create an extension of your auric field through your fingertips. (This involves all of the original 13 rays.)
- Place your hands/fingers upon the body section needing healing. A vortex (a center of energy which is transformative) is created within this area from the swirling 13 rays.
- One hand's vortex is spinning clockwise (typically the right hand) and the other hand is spinning counter-clockwise (typically the left hand). [This is the balance of male/female energy.]
- Imagine a healthy body part; visualize <u>a perfect blue-print</u> superimposing itself over the organ or area being healed.
- You may add sound or "toning" to address the tissues.
- As with any healing technique, be sure to clear and ground when completed.

Note: It is a good idea to work in threes (male and female healers forming a triad).

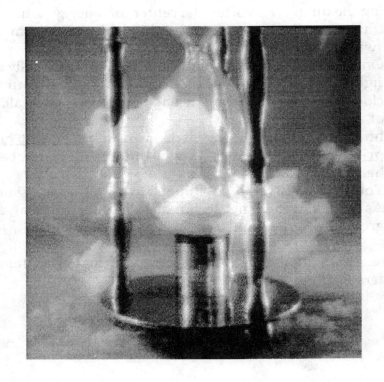

Chapter 25

Advanced Psi Arts

====

*"Time and space are modes
by which we think,
not conditions in which we live."*

---*Albert Einstein*

As your command of energy intensifies, as your willingness to clear and align all parts of yourself continues, and as your spiritual journey towards Oneness becomes the most important thing in the world, you may begin to notice strange yet wonderful bodily phenomena occurring. They are the *psi arts*, or what has been commonly termed "paranormal phenomena."

Numerous abilities* fall into this category including but not limited to: telepathy, clairvoyance, clairaudience, clairsentience, materialization of objects, psychokinesis, and bilocation. For the purpose of this book, I will only cover in-depth, teleportation, levitation, invisibility, and shapeshifting.

The biggest obstacles to succeeding in the psi arts are part of what I call the FUD factor: *fear, uncertainty,* and *doubt*. When this factor dominates you, it invalidates your experience; your desires become unattainable. This truth manifests as a mask of false humbleness, imbalanced self-esteem. The FUD factor acts as a deterrent to realized spiritual attainment. *Maya*, or illusion, is always willing to support your personal view of self as a limited, unworthy being.

Like the ascended masters, you are capable of Self-awareness; you can grasp the underlying cosmic laws that govern the time/space continuum, a system set up for our own protection. Its design prevents us from going to the end of the story before we fully understand the nature of multiple "reality".

You would not want anything less than full illumination, complete self-realization. You can learn the psi arts along the way without sacrificing your goal.

---

* For those who are interested, there are many reference books available on these subjects.

Personally, I have spiritual teachers who chose to ascend from this physical 3rd plane while concurrently developing the side gifts. They give the psi arts no excess importance in the scheme of things. There are others who say it is a distraction along the spiritual path. I honor that perspective as well, for I have seen some talented people fall by the wayside, or lose valuable ground. However, most of them "fell" long before the psi arts were attained. They lost their focus to one or more of the four pitfalls: fear, alter ego, greed, and adultery. They also exhibited an unwillingness to align their fragmented inner child or other unaligned aspects of themselves; they resisted dealing with imbalance in any of their four bodies.

I choose to give you access to the development of the psi arts rather than censor them or drive them further into secret mystery schools, available only a chosen few. It is time to bring these divine gifts out into the open; they can play an important part in the glorious new dawn of planetary awakening! Those who use them to control others, or have less than stellar reasons for utilizing them, will probably not manifest them fully or lose them soon enough.

Teleportation

Teleportation is defined as the act of moving physical matter from one place to another, often through "solid" matter. It can also involve moving from one plane to another, moving from one parallel dimension to another, or even one time period to another. The common ingredient is the instantaneous movement of the entire physical body from one space to another.

There are numerous documented cases of teleportation, many spontaneous in nature. Explanation eludes investigators; most have chosen to place this uncommon phenomenon in the "odd, unexplained" file. A plausible reason for sudden unplanned teleportation could be the effect that the earth's ley lines or vortices play in distorting the time/space continuum, allowing for the physical body to suddenly shift in density. One's body then behaves like sub-atomic particles documented in the study of quantum physics; particles that can be instantaneously somewhere else.

Another reason for teleportation--or for that matter, levitation and the other psi arts--could be that those adepts who have come to comprehend the illusory nature of matter have accepted the plausibility of this process as being purely natural, and not particularly mysterious. It is a God-given ability, albeit latent in most humankind, available to us all with practice.*

Several alleged, well-known teleporters, past and present, include Count Saint Germain of 18th century Europe, Babaji of the Himalayas, Sister Mary of Agreda, Padre Pio of Italy, and Satya Sai Baba of India; there are many other lesser known adepts of this art. What distinguishes them from the spontaneous teleporters is their master-level spiritual enlightenment. Spiritual devotion is always their first priority and the bodily shifts occur as a natural by-product. There is a conscious command over the experience that comes to them as they master teleportation. Their planned destination is consciously induced. These enlightened beings prove to us that the psi arts are not

---

*As I stated in Chapter 4, we carry many undeveloped neurons in our brains, contained within the *tensor*, or psychic center. Long ago, the human *tensor* mutated due to planetary traumas, and limited thinking.

only possible, but probable. These gifts are emerging quite naturally in the New Age of quantum awareness.

Teleportation Exercise

Purpose: To understand the fluidity of matter. To stretch your boundary of limited experience to one of unlimited perspective. To increase your wisdom and connection to the One.

Notes: When you teleport between planes as a physical essence, memory of where you've been, or what you've experienced, is not always strong, at first. The journey is similar to a veiled "past" lifetime amnesia-state of consciousness. Extensive details will not be easily accessible. Eventually, with repetition of the teleportation experience you will cultivate a way of remembering. Atomic structural changes take place within the physical body when it travels between dimensions. However, the original body's *blueprint* is always re-established upon your return. One can teleport in the unconscious sleep-state,* with little or no memory, or consciously through meditation, with easier recall.

Teleporting on the earthly plane can be used to help others in a healing or supportive way. It also offers a chance to gain insight and wisdom, and can be used as a vehicle for channeling the Love and Light of the Source.

Remember, the state of teleportation includes taking the whole body with you. It is *not* an out-of-body state.

---

* You can treat your sleep-time excursions as you would *lucid dreaming*, by writing down your memories upon awakening in an ongoing dream journal.

Procedure:

- Ground, clear, balance, and protect with a strong, protective shield of your choosing.
- You may facilitate the process with the use of rose essential oil. It has a very uplifting affect. Apply it directly under the nose, or add some rose oil to an aromatherapy diffuser in your meditation space.
- Compact your chakras into one location. Link to the Sun and Moon through a chakra braid made up of all 13 color rays.
- Link a chakra braid to all five of the elements: earth, air, water, fire, and ether.
- When a conscious teleportation experience occurs, you will feel as though you are being energetically stretched across the distance of a mile. You will feel pulled from the front, while simultaneously being drawn from the back. You will physically "disappear" from normal vision. You may also experience vibration within your body, as though you've become a loud motor. The experience is not unpleasant, unless fear overtakes you. Don't worry; you will return intact, with all of your body parts in the right place! You have simply stepped up your vibratory rate, and temporarily shifted physical matter to a more tenuous frequency.
- As you enter a tunnel of energy, you will rapidly propel through space, usually at the speed of light. You may enter a wormhole, or teleport outside the bounds of a wormhole. You will stretch the boundaries of your physical matter as though it were composed of a fluid substance, instead of dense flesh and bone.
- During a sleep-time teleportation you will not feel any bodily effects. You may wake-up feeling a little different, not as physically grounded. To know for sure that you've physically teleported, someone would have had to observe your "disappearance and reappearance." You may remember bits and fragments of the experi-

ence which you could confirm with your spirit guide during meditation.

• Upon completion of a teleportation you will find yourself back home in a normal physical state.

• Ground, ground, and ground again! If you are still too "spacey" disconnect from the five elements, and the Sun and Moon. (These links would automatically dissipate after a time anyway.)

Levitation

Levitation is defined as the state of floating or arising above ground, defying the law of gravity. During the levitation state, anti-gravity has manifested for a time. Levitation is often accompanied by extreme states of meditative bliss and a heightened connection to God.

The art of levitation has been documented for hundreds of years. Sometimes levitation appears as a spontaneous, unplanned, total surprise to the levitated one. Most other levitations seem to be meditatively and spiritually generated, usually experienced by mystics and yogis in a high state of ecstatic communion with the Divine. Some past well known levitators include Italy's St. Theresa of Avila, Lahiri Mahasaya of India and St. Thomas Aquinas.

Transcendental Meditation (TM) reportedly teaches how to achieve the levitation state through contemplation. Other methods are taught by mystery schools or yogic orders. Some adepts receive the information directly from Spirit.

Levitation Exercise

Purpose: To understand the nature of anti-gravity, and to lose the heaviness of physical matter. To bring one closer to understanding the mastery of *pranayama* (control of one's life-force). **This is not a circus trick or a trivial attention-getter.**

Procedure:
- Ground, clear, balance, and protect with a strong, protective energy shield.
- Compact the chakras to one location. Construct a braid out of the 13 color rays and link it directly to the Moon, Sun, and a planet of heavy gravitational force, such as Jupiter or Saturn.
- Practice! Remember the delusionary nature of the FUD factor.
- Don't be discouraged if levitation has not occurred. You are elevating your consciousness every time you practice it. As with any technique, it will manifest when the timing is perfect and not one moment before.
- Regardless of the outcome, be sure to re-ground. Not reconnecting to the earth will make you very out-of-touch with your physical body, possibly dangerous to yourself and others because of your ungroundedness.
- Clear all braids.

Invisibility

Purpose: To master the physical plane vibration. To truly know that you are composed of refined frequency and that matter is only a thought of the Divine Being. *Only practice this technique with the utmost integrity and respect for the Cosmic Order.*

Procedure:
- Wrap yourself in an energy shield* of your own choosing.
- Ground to the earth. Let the excess energy dissipate.
- Invoke the three elements of *water*, *air*, and *ether*.
- Compact all of your chakras to your base center. Send a link composed of all 13 color rays into the earth.
- From the base chakra, bring forth a braided triad of *clear*, *gold*, and *silver* energy, and link it to the elements ether, air, and water.
- Practice, practice, practice! Surrender has a lot to do with success when it comes to this and all techniques.
- Invisibility will occur only when you are ready to handle it.
- When you've completed this technique, ground and re-balance your chakras, as always.

---

* An energy shield is a form of invisibility by its very nature. Wrapping yourself in various force fields keeps you from being "seen" by the observer.

Shapeshifting

The phenomenon of *shapeshifting* is a magical, shamanic process. It allows you to move your physical being into a different vibrational energy--generally an animal form.

One shapeshifts to expand one's concept of *being*. We do this by honoring the intelligence, wisdom, love, resourcefulness, and multiple other gifts that stem from nearby sentient kingdoms. Shapeshifting shows us in the most direct way that we are intrinsically connected to all of the living organisms in our cosmic tapestry.

In this particular book, I will not be including a specific technique on shapeshifting. I only teach shapeshifting to students who have reached the "master color healer" level in my hands-on classes. The knowledge and secrets of shapeshifting will come to you as you evolve as a healer. Should you attempt shapeshifting at some future point in time, the following suggestions are important and worth remembering:

1. Attempt to shapeshift in the company of someone you trust, a friend who understands and can facilitate the process.
2. Before you begin, make sure that you've protected, grounded, balanced, and cleared all four of your bodies. If you are in a state of physical, emotional, mental, or spiritual crisis, this would <u>not</u> be the time to practice the art of shapeshifting.
3. Be specific regarding which animal you intend to shapeshift into. Start with one of your animal totems, eventually graduating to one of your own "past" lives.
4. This ability can help you to make great strides towards clearing your physical, emotional, and mental bodies.

The Quantum Dimensions--24 to 33

A short while after receiving data on the new *shadow* levels of existence, an additional set of dimensions made themselves known to me. I choose to call them the *quantum dimensions*. They are a balance of male and female polarities.

NOTE: The triads of alchemical rays may create a color that's a bit unexpected. In some cases certain rays of the triad may be dominant; that is, existing in greater concentrations over the other one or two rays contained within the triad.

- Balance your chakras. Connect them to the Earth, Sun, and Moon.
- Combine your chakras to one spot, either the base or the crown.
- Send all 13 rays out from that chakra point to the **24th Dimension**. It is a symbolic registry of the masculine and feminine, the god and goddess. It wavers between visibility and invisibility because it is on the edge of the color spectrum. It was created by an alchemical triad of color energy consisting of *translucent blue*, *green*, and *orange*, which formed a **rust red** color. Its symbol is the **Star of David** (a triangle overlaid with an inverted triangle).
- Unlink your chakra connection to the 24th Dimension and re-link to the **25th Dimension**. This plane is a vibrational level where beings appear and disappear; one moment they are physical while in the next they are non-physical. The 25th level is composed of radio waves rather than light waves. This gives it a shimmering, glowing appearance. There is a wide variety of orange and yellow colors, along with some reds. The

alchemical triad of color energy that created this level was *orange*, *yellow*, and *red*, forming **pumpkin** color. The symbol for this dimension is a **lighted candle**.

- Unlink your chakra connection to the 25th Dimension and re-link it to the ***26th Dimension***. This plane has strong, pleasant odors of food, though none is ever eaten at this level. Clear is the only color seen at this plane. The alchemical color triad that created this dimension was *clear*, *white*, and *gold*, which formed a **moonstone** color. Its symbol is a **cup**. *The 26th plane of existence is directly connected to the Source energy on the 13th and 33rd Dimensions.*

- Unlink your chakra connection to the 26th Dimension and re-link it to the ***27th Dimension***. This plane looks like a crystal planet. (It is similar to Galaton, another planet in an adjoining universe.) There are many crystalline forms here of varying bright colors. The 27th Dimension radiates joy, bordering on euphoria. The alchemical color triad that created this dimension was *rose*, *purple*, and *red*, which formed a **mauve** color. The symbol for this plane is a **single-terminated quartz crystal**.

- Unlink your chakra connection to the 27th Dimension and re-link it to the ***28th Dimension***. This is a dimension filled with "extinct" lifeforms, such as lions with bird feet, birds with 40 foot wing spans, and dinosaurs. These beings are not carnivorous. There is much harmony on the 28th plane and no burdens. The alchemical color triad that created this level was *yellow*, *orange*, and *green*, which formed a **goldenrod** color. The symbol for this plane is the **inverted pyramid**.

- Unlink your chakra connection to the 28th Dimension and re-link it to the ***29th Dimension***. This plane is exclusively shaded with the rose ray. This plane also carries the subtle scent of rose. It is a soft dimension; objects "feel" similar to foam rubber. The alchemical color triad that formed this plane was *rose*, *red*, and *white*, forming a **rose** color. The symbol for this plane is the **rose**.

- Unlink your chakra connection to the 29th Dimension and re-link it to the **30th Dimension**. This plane appears to have no human beings, and few plants or animals. It contains fire and ice which never combine to form water. The colors red, orange, yellow, and blue dominate this level of existence. It is a plane of ideas. The alchemical color triad that created this plane was *orange*, *yellow*, and *translucent blue*, which formed a **khaki green** color. The symbol for this plane is a **chalice**.

- Unlink your chakra connection to the 30th Dimension and re-link it to the **31st Dimension**. This plane looks like Swiss cheese. It contains many interdimensional holes; when you enter one hole, you come out someplace else on this dimension. There is an emphasis on the colors silver, gold, and black. The alchemical color triad that created this plane was *silver*, *black* and *gold*, which formed **electrum** (a silver gold color). The symbol for this plane is a **squiggly line** that looks like a worm.

- Unlink your chakra connection to the 31st Dimension and re-link it to the *32nd Dimension*. This plane is very gaseous in nature . Its colors are muted. Beings appear as specters as their images "come" and "go". They are ascetics choosing to remain in trance or in the out-of-body state. The alchemical color triad that created this plane was *green*, *violet*, and *clear*, which formed the dual colors of **violet surrounded on its outer edge by green**. The symbol for this plane is a **teardrop** with a violet interior and a green exterior.

- Unlink your chakra connection to the 32nd Dimension and re-link it to the *33rd Dimension*. This plane is very mountainous with many bright, shiny colors. If a question were asked aloud here, one would not hear an echo, one would hear an answer. It is the *oracle* plane. My guides tell me that this is where Moses transformed himself when he "climbed the mountain." The alchemical color triad that created this plane was *gold*, *red*, and *black*, which formed a **copper** color. The symbol for this plane is **a cross with a crown within it**. *This dimension is directly connected to the Source energy, found within the 26th and the 13th dimensions.*

- Unlink your chakra connection to the 33rd Dimension. Dissipate all extra energy. Re-ground to the earth.

Dimension	Symbol	Ray Colors
24th	Star of David	Blue, Green, Orange
25th	Candle	Orange, Yellow, Red
26th	Cup	Clear , White, Gold
27th	Quartz crystal	Rose, Purple, Red
28th	Inverted pyramid	Yellow, Orange, Green

Dimension	Symbol	Ray Colors
29th	Rose	Rose, Red, White
30th	Chalice	Orange, Yellow, Blue
31st	Squiggly Line	Silver, Black, Gold
32nd	Teardrop	Green, Violet, Clear
33rd	Crown	Gold, Red, Black

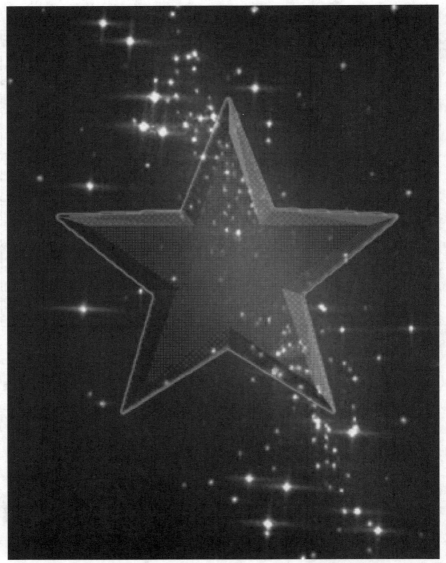

Sarah Steinbach

Epilogue

The Emerald Star

The Emerald Star

From the heart of the emerald
Through the dimensional mists

To heal, to align
To balance, to bless

The eternal star
The emerald dance.

—Althea
December 1991

309

Once upon a time, at the 12th dimensional level, an idea was conceived regarding an arrangement of energies that would encompass healing. This configuration of energies was a blueprint for what would later be known as the *Emerald Star*.

The care of this blueprint of energies was entrusted to the Green Ray, who kept it safe and maintained its integrity.

As time went on, Creation became denser as it expanded out into multiple levels of vibration; the duality of physical existence within the Milky Way galaxy (on the 3rd dimension) became fraught with chaos and disharmony. There were those who desired to rule over others with an autocratic form of government. These leaders, as well as many of their followers, lost sight of their own divinity and their symbiotic interdependence with one another. There were several galactic wars, each more horrifying than the last, as each emperor's army found new ways to eliminate those who would rebel against their authority.

It seemed as though all hope was lost, along with countless lives. But there always remained those brave souls with farsighted vision who never lost their connection to the One. Many of them lost their lives for their truth. Their vision of a brotherhood and sisterhood rooted in the One kept them strong.

Eventually, the majority of humanity grew weary of the relentless fighting and its unsatisfying results. The last of the galactic wars drew to a conclusion. There remained a group of beings who had attained self-mastery, who remembered the healing energies entrusted to the Green Ray. It was determined that it was time to bring forth those energies onto a physical dimension, to offer hope and healing, to bring Love and Light once again to a struggling humanity.

The founders of the Emerald Star housed their order on an unattractive planet, one in which the existing galactic empire had no interest. It was located in the constellation of the Southern Cross, on the outer edges of the known universe. Healing data was stored in underground, underwater secret caverns to avoid attracting attention from the Empire. Those dedicated to the preservation of precious knowledge guarded it carefully.

The data included information regarding magnetics, miscellaneous types of bodywork, crystal and herbal healing, and color energy techniques. It described the importance of balance within the human vehicle and the attainment of alignment among the four bodies (physical, emotional, mental, and spiritual). It gave responsibility for one's own health back to one's own self, not to others. It explained how to be more in tune with the Source and It's creation through the understanding that we are undifferentiated from the very radiant energy that we channel in the healing process.

When the last treaty had been signed by warring factions within the galaxy, it became safe for the Emerald Star to surface. It eventually moved its main facility to a planet within the constellation of Altair. Representatives of this healing order spread to existing dimensions.

After a number of years of peaceful coexistence, the 3rd Dimension--of the post galactic war time period--progressed spiritually to the point where it collectively made a vibrational shift to what we know of at this time as the current 4th dimension.

Many representatives of the Emerald Star healing association are currently upon this 3rd plane of existence. As humanity awakens upon this dimension, we will become more open to the data and the help that this collective offers. Bygone days of the galaxy have taught those within the Emerald Star that patience pays. "The true believer begins with himself."

Afterword

No Limits

Do not fear, there is no limit
The promise has been granted;
We are part of the Infinite
The old images were slanted.
Those false views are corrected
And now given this new Light
Everyone is connected!
This new journey is a joy, not a fight;
So accept this, be gifted.
Rejoice,
The veils have been lifted.
Give voice
As you teleport to destinations far
And as you see that energy, time, and matter
Have escaped this belljar.

----Adassan
April 1995

Having completed your reading and practiced the exercises in this book, you are ready to begin to apply what you've learned to your life path. Unless you intimately experience these techniques (or other powerful spiritual exercises) in your own life as a positive means of growth, you will not be able to effectively transfer their full healing power and essence to the recipient.

When you live in the physical world variety of experience is a gift. It helps one attain the highest level of experience. You cannot easily shift something without the personal experience of it. **Knowledge without wisdom ultimately means little.** It is difficult to attain wisdom without experience.

Now, I'm not stating that you should experience drugs, spousal abuse, or other forms of hard learning, because without these experiences you cannot help someone who has been in that "school of hard knocks." What I am conveying is the idea that as you have lived multiple lives on this 3rd plane Earth playground, you will have experienced failure, deprivation, hate, envy, resentment, misunderstanding, and many other forms of learning. You have also experienced their inverse: success, abundance, love, kindness, harmony, and understanding. Arguably, you may have learned more from the former set of life challenges than the latter gifts, but they enriched your life beyond measure. See them as a tool for growth, self-acceptance, self-empowerment, and alignment with the God-self within you.

So many of us forget *why* we are here, and what we are here to accomplish. The root causes of this are fear and unworthiness; they create forgetfulness regarding our true nature. Remember, you *always* create your own reality. If you don't like what you have created, it is time to change it around.

I hope you realize that you, as the healer, do not *really* "heal" the client. You present a mirror to him or her to show imbalance. You help the recipient move back into a state of balance and wholeness by reflecting wholeness back to the client.

To do this, the color therapist needs to be able not only to transfer the harmonizing energy of Creation, but to reflect this energy in his or her own life to as great a degree as possible.

All of us, designated healers and non-healers alike, are in a constant, albeit shifting, state of being. Our lives exemplify healing, for until we are in a state of perfection, our life's journey is one of healing our fears, limits, blocks, and general imbalances. You could say that the healer exemplifies the classic archetype of the "Wounded Healer." The wounded healer participates in the healing process with the wounded recipient, and understands that they are co-creating states of balance for them both. It would not be considered unusual or strange if you find many of your clients with the same physical, emotional, mental, and spiritual challenges as yourself. In helping them to heal the affliction, you will have the opportunity to heal it within yourself.

To exemplify integrity as a healer is not to force clients to clear or heal. If they don't feel safe with a healer, they will shut down or find it difficult to make positive shifts. Some healers attempt to force the process, unable to allow for a client's individuality, or unwilling to look like a "failure" if a recipient doesn't appear to heal. Remember that a personal commitment has to be made to *change* a pattern, even after the pattern is moved energetically by you in the healing process. Operate with a non-linear mode of facilitation, accepting that each person is unique. **Hold the intent of wholeness by being more observant than treatment-motivated.**

I have previously touched on *the shadow self* and the necessity to align and integrate it within you. This process of validating your shadow self's existence takes a lot of courage on your part. This is where we lose many people along the path of self-realization; this is a step that cannot be side-stepped or shortchanged in your process. It takes a deep level of honesty to deal with one's shortcomings, to embrace all parts of yourself, positive or negative. Do not polarize yourself. *Anything that forms separateness creates resistance and non-acceptance, contributing to a mutation process.* You are both Light and Dark, as is Creation. Accepting this fact fully brings illumination, and a conscious decision to completely embrace your divinity.

May you enjoy fulfilling hours transmitting the healing energies of radiant color to all who desire these vibrations. May you become ever more aligned with your own Higher Self and Oversoul. The willingness to channel wisdom and healing helps us to be more open to the energy of the Oversoul. We often have fears and feelings of hurt and rejection. By opening to Love or refined frequency, we wipe away obstacles to experiencing the love of self, and then, by extension, the process of loving others. May you truly *know* that you are Pure Essence, as is your Father-Mother God. You are spirit beings cloaked in biological dress, here to bridge physical with non-physical, matter with anti-matter, time with no-time. By your absolute knowingness that you *are* Source, have *always been* Source, and *will forever* be Source, you will find yourself remaining strong, constant, and unaffected through the many challenging, radically shifting days to come.

Let your life exemplify the blended diversity, complete empowerment, and Source-connected harmony of the Rainbow.

Alijandra
San Jose, CA
April 1995

Glossary of Terms

A

Akashic Records The cosmic library where all data that has ever been thought or done is stored. Is accessible through intuitive means.

Alchemical Rays The blending together of rays that have formed a compound; this blending modifies the structure, making it nearly impossible to separate the fundamental elements.

Alchemy A tool for transformation, both physical (turning lead into gold), as well as, psychological or spiritual (taking one to cosmic states of awareness).

Alignment The state of being balanced in our 4 bodies (physical, emotional, mental, and spiritual).

Anti-Gravity Gravity which pushes *up* rather than *down*. Considered a *negative space*.

Anti-Matter The same as *matter*, but carries the opposite electrical charge.

Aura Any electromagnetic field of energy that surrounds living beings. Contains color, as well as, symbols. Is impacted by the current states of the four bodies.

B

Black Hole Collapsed stars in which no light can escape from the star's enormous gravitational field. A gateway to parallel universes and openings to warps in the fabric of time.

Blended Rays The energies of two or more rays that are blended together to create a *composite* energy, or mixture. They can still be distilled from the composite blend.

Body Scan The process of intuitively perceiving healing data by moving one's hands along the edge of a person's auric field.

Braid *Three* or more links of energy or rays that are woven together to a particular point, or vortex, with another essence.

C

Camouflaged Energy Matching the energy of another's auric field in terms of color for reasons either positive or non-positive.

Causal Plane A non-physical, inner plane of Mind, wherein you create your own reality.

Cellular Footprint A non-physical energy grid composed of elemental crystals and gemstones that is placed around a person for the purpose of protection.

Chakra Energy center in the body where a concentration of nerves congregate; a particular gland, organ, and level of consciousness is associated with each chakra.

Chalice A spiritual symbol dating back to ancient times. The metaphysical meaning is a symbolic container for holding the most purified alchemical essence.

Channel To become a vehicle for the flow of cosmic energy through healing or dissemination of truth.

Chiron A planetoid orbiting between Saturn and Uranus, discovered in 1977. Astrologically, it is called the "rainbow bridge between the inner and outer planets" by author Barbara Hand Clow.

Clearing Dissolving the blockages to growth while harmonizing and balancing all four bodies, allowing the alignment of the bodies.

Clairaudience The intuitive art of *hearing* beyond what society considers "normal" auditory input. This can involve auditory perception of spiritual guides and counsel, or sounds outside of "normal" perception.

Clairsentience The intuitive art of *feeling* subtleties such as auric fields, multiple probabilities, and realities beyond what society considers "normal."

Clairvoyance   The intuitive art of *seeing* auric fields, multiple probabilities, and realities beyond the visual perception of what society considers "normal."

Color Healing/Color Therapy   The application of multidimensional frequencies of Light to balance, heal, elevate, link with more refined energies and beings, and to connect with the Source.

Crystallization Process   Shifting the body's vibrations to a more refined and amplified state of energy by psychically placing points of crystalline frequency at sensing/transmitting areas of the body.

Ɛ

Electromagnetic Energy   The balance of yin-yang (female/male) within the auric field of a living essence.

Emerald Star   A multi-level cosmic healing order, composed of general medical practitioners, where several styles of holistic healing practices occur.

Empath   A being who is able to become "one" with another person to such an extent that he/she feels exactly what the other is feeling.

Energy   Vital or life force. An aspect of the Radiant One's unlimited emanations.

Energy Block   Location in one's essence where a "roadblock" or wall is placed. Energy cannot flow well or move past this point.

Essence   A living force or intelligence that has a soul.

G

Gaia   The spiritual consciousness of planet Earth.

H

Halls of Amente   The sacred, inner Earth where Earth's history is stored; the *soul* of the planet resides there.

Harmonic Convergence   Cosmic event that heralded revolutionary shift in consciousness. It occurred on August 16th and 17th, 1987, and signaled the end of the materialistic cycle. Coined by Jose Arguelles, its occurrence was based on the Mayan calendar as well as other corroborating sources (Hopi, Aztec, astrological, and New Age) which set same dates. It was the start of major planetary *clearing* processes.

Healing   That process where one creates a safe place for another individual so that they can attune themselves to their own personal alignment.

Healer   A facilitator who assists someone with bringing forth his/her own powers of recuperation with a goal to balance them in wellness.

Higher Self   That part of your essence (at the spiritual level) that links you with all other dimensional parts of yourself and connects you with the Over-soul. [A good analogy would be a computer terminal which is linked to the mainframe.]

Holistic/Wholistic Seeing the body as a whole with each part connected to the other.

Holographic   A multidimensional perspective of reality which teaches that all Creation is a part of the Whole, or *One*.

Hyperspace   Embraces multiple concepts of the time/space continuum explained by quantum physics.

I

Interdimension/Multidimension   The many different levels of existence beyond our five senses and view of this 3rd plane reality.

Inner Child   One's childhood aspect which always remains alive, no matter what age is attained. Needs to be aligned with the adult self for full self-realization or enlightenment.

Instantaneity An altering of the time/space continuum wherein a form of teleportation is involved.

Invisibility The practice of being able to quicken one's vibration to such an extent that one would disappear to normal human eyesight.

K

Karma This is the universal law of "cause and effect" or balance.

Kirlian Photography The process of capturing on film the electro-magnetic resonance surrounding a living being.

Kundalini Hindu word for the life-force energy originating at the base chakra. In an "awakened" state, it spirals the spinal column upward to the crown chakra.

L

Levitation The psychic art of lightening the density of the physical body so that it defies the law of gravity.

Ley Line Electromagnetic lines that crisscross the earth below (physical) and above the earth (non-physical) to form a grid. These lines are connected to vortices.

Lightworker An evolved person who is committed to the growth of self and the wellness of all living beings on his/her planetary home. Also known as a *Rainbow Warrior*.

M

Montecillio The etheric "city," or spiritual blueprint, for the ancient continent of Lemuria.

Movement Anti-stagnation. The force needed for growth.

Multidimension/Interdimension The many different levels of existence beyond our five senses and view of this 3rd plane reality.

O

Out-of-Body Experience The ability to *consciously*, temporarily, exit the physical body for the purpose of experiencing other worlds or dimensions.

Oversoul The original energy from which you and others split after moving from the Creator. There are multiple oversouls in Creation.

P

Parallel Universes Multiple realities, *mirror images* of our own universe.

Psychic Hook Usually attached without conscious permission, it is an energy link to another person for the purpose of fearfully holding on, or for the draining of their energy.

Psychic Surgery Intense healing by physical penetration through the painless parting of the molecular structure of the body with minimal loss of blood, or energetic penetration of the body.

Pulsar Is formed from neutron stars rotating around each other in an opposing dance attraction and repulsion. Huge amounts of heat and light are generated by this object, along with a strong, intense surges of gravity and magnetism.

Q

Quantum Dimensions The dimensions labeled 24 through 33 which carry both the negative and positive polarities.

Quasars Quasi-stellar objects. The most luminous in the universe, they shine with the equivalent radiance of a hundred galaxies.

ℝ

Rainbow Rays Commonly refers to the "original" 13 rays of Creation. However, they also include the rays that have evolved into *blended* and *alchemical* combinations.

Rainbow Warriors Individuals of different races, cultures, and economic backgrounds who have unique abilities to communicate as "beacons of Light." Otherwise known as *lightworkers*.

Responsibility *The ability to respond.* The willingness to acknowledge and claim one's own involvement and action in everything that happens to him/her rather than blame another. *Response vs. reaction.*

S

Sentience Capable of consciousness; has a soul essence.

Shadow Dimensions The "unseen" levels that comprise the dimensions 14 through 23. They vibrate with the negative (feminine) polarity.

Shambhala The etheric "city," or spiritual blueprint, for the ancient continent of Atlantis.

Shangri-La The etheric "city," or spiritual blueprint, for the ancient continent of Sumeria.

Shapeshifting   The process of shifting one's energy to embody that of an animal totem or a *past* lifetime.

Shield   A spiritual symbol of protection.   Also called "medicine shield."

Simultaneous Lifetimes   The understanding that seeing our *past* and *future* lifetimes also exist in the Eternal Now or present reality.

Source/Womb   God, the Supreme Intelligence or Presence. Where Creation was birthed.

Sword   A spiritual symbol of power used for intuitive discernment and protection. Cuts out things you no longer need.

Symbiotic   Energies blending in harmony and balance.

𝒯

Tao   The Void of Creation, or the Source.

Telepathy   A psi art that expresses mind-to-mind, not with verbal or written communication.

Teleportation   The psi ability to instantly transport oneself from one locale to another through solid matter.

Time Rip/Time Warp   A "wrinkle", or distortion, in time.

Time Travel The ability to travel backward or forward in the time/space continuum.

Time Vault Power spots on the earth where the ancients stored valuable, advanced data before the collapse of their civilizations.

V

Void Described in the Tao as the eternal blackness.

Vortex/Vortices Concentrations of energy. May be electric (yang energy), magnetic (yin energy), or electromagnetic (both yin and yang) in resonance.

W

Walk-In A soul or Higher Self entering a physical body as an exchange of souls during the course of a lifetime. (A prior agreement rather than a possession.) Generally, a highly evolved soul who wishes to do service in this lifetime by completing a mission for the benefit of humankind.

Walk-Out The soul essence leaving a physical body in the soul exchange process. Either feels his/her life mission is accomplished or does not feel able to go further with the physical expression.

White Brotherhood   A fraternal order of spiritual essences who were originally tied to the Earth karmic wheel and ascended to other planes of existence.

White Hole   Has evolved from a black hole with sufficient energy force to overcome its gravitation or mass, then spews out light, color, and information. A white hole can be on the other side of a black hole, however, it is more likely a black hole running "backward" in time.   (An anti-gravity universe.)

Wholistic/Holistic   Seeing the body as a whole with each part connected to the other.

Womb/Source   God, the Supreme Intelligence or Presence. Where Creation was birthed.

Wormholes   Cosmic "highways" connecting planetary bodies or parallel universes.

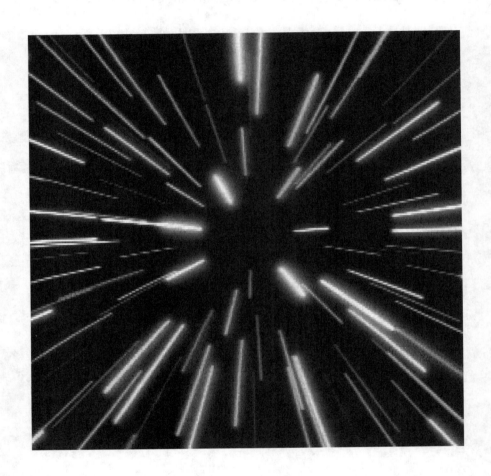

Ordering Information

For additional books, information on classes, tapes, or videos, and/or to be placed on Alijandra's mailing list, contact:

Emerald Star Publishing
P. O. Box 32818
San Jose, California 95152-2818
(800) 395-5811 or (408) 986-8550

❑ Send information on *Rainbow Rays* color classes and lectures

❑ Send information regarding other *Emerald Star Publishing* products (audio, video, etc.)

❑ Send additional copies of <u>Healing with the Rainbow Rays</u>

Quantity: _____ @ $18.95 per copy $ _____

CA residents add $1.38 sales tax per book $ _____

Postage and handling $ _____
($2.00 per book in USA/$5.00 per book outside USA)
TOTAL ENCLOSED $ _____

<u>*Method of payment*</u> (circle one)
Check/Money Order   MasterCard   Visa

credit card # _____

expiration date: month _____ year _____

Signature: _____

Name: _____

Address: _____

City: _____ State: _____ Zip:_____

Phone: (_____) _____